What Are Stem Cells?

RHETORIC, CULTURE, AND SOCIAL CRITIQUE

SERIES EDITOR
John Louis Lucaites

What Are Stem Cells?

Definitions at the Intersection of Science and Politics

JOHN LYNCH

THE UNIVERSITY OF ALABAMA PRESS
Tuscaloosa

Typeface: Bembo

∞
The paper on which this book is printed meets the minimum requirements of American
National Standard for Information Sciences—Permanence of Paper for Printed Library
Materials, ANSI Z39.48-1984.

Library of Congress Cataloging-in-Publication Data

Lynch, John (John Alexander), 1976–
    What are stem cells? : definitions at the intersection of science and politics / John Lynch.
        p. cm. — (Rhetoric, culture, and social critique)
    Includes bibliographical references and index.
    ISBN 978-0-8173-1748-5 (cloth : alk. paper) — ISBN 978-0-8173-8576-7 (electronic)
  1. Stem cells. 2. Reasoning. 3. Stem cells—Social aspects. 4. Stem cells—Moral and ethical
aspects. I. Title.
    QH588.S83L96 2011
    616′.02774—dc22
                                                                                    2011003386

Cover image: © Krishnacreations | Dreamstime.com

Contents

Acknowledgments

This project is the result of serendipity as much as it is the result of any intention on my part. It began with an interest in science and an inability to do well in math—despite the best efforts of my accountant father and math teacher mother—which led through a circuitous path to graduate studies in the rhetoric of science. This specific project on stem cells resulted from an off-hand suggestion by my advisor after an entirely different project died on the vine. Without that initial suggestion to "check out stem cell research" and then substantial amounts of support and guidance over the years since, this project would have never happened. For that, I deeply thank my mentor Celeste Condit.

Other mentors and colleagues also deserve considerable thanks. Victoria Davion, Kevin DeLuca, Tom Lessl, John Murphy, and Steve Stice read the original version of this project. Jeff Bennett and Leah Ceccarelli have generously offered advice about the publication process. Gail Fairhurst and Judith Trent kindly read through grant proposals and offered suggestions for the grant and the book project, and Teresa Sabourin has been a supportive department chair.

I would also like to thank the graduate students who ably assisted in transcribing and keeping track of the television news media examined in this book. Adam Godfrey, Cecilia Holmes, and Katie Sayers were all amazingly helpful.

Finally, I want to thank my families of blood and of choice: my parents, John and Karen Lynch; my sister, Jill Atwood, and her daughters, Brynn and Katelyn; Jeremy and Lisa Boerger for being good friends and for making me the godfather to their three children, Stephen, RJ, and Ilsa. Most of all, I want to thank my partner, John Baughcum, for his constant love and considerable patience with my foibles.

The media portion of this project was supported by a University Research Council summer fellowship from the University of Cincinnati in 2007. Parts of chapters 3 and 4 appeared in my article "Stem Cells and the Embryo: Biorhetoric and Scientism in Congressional Debate" in *Public Understandings of Science* 18, pages 309–324.

1
Science-Based Controversies
and Idioms of Public Argument

In August 2000, PBS's *NewsHour* aired a debate on embryonic stem (ES) cells. The representatives of the two sides—Richard Doerflinger, from the United States Conference of Catholic Bishops, and Daniel Perry, chairman of the Patients' Coalition for Urgent Research—took little time highlighting what they saw as the core issues in stem cell research. According to Doerflinger, "For the first time in federal history, U.S. History, the federal government will actually be taking a class of human beings, a form of developing human life which is what even the NIH calls these embryos, and destroying that life for the benefit of others." For Doerflinger, the creation of embryonic stem cells destroys human life, an action even more troubling because scientists could alternatively obtain stem cells from adults without the loss of life. For Perry, in contrast, the issue is creating effective therapies for cancer and Parkinson's disease. Adult stem cells do not work: "Even after all of these years, we have not been able to make adult stem cells replace potentially, any cell in the body. That's the great promise of embryonic stem cells. . . . How can we tell a young woman, diabetic at age 20, we're going to wait five years and just study adult stem cells and we may say, well that didn't work, now we're going to try something else—when in the meantime, she may have faced the loss of sight, amputation, kidney failure? I think it would be immoral and unconscionable to tell patients wait until first we try this avenue that so far has not proven effective." It is unsurprising that a spokesperson for the Catholic Church opposes scientific experiments that involve the earliest stages of human life and that an advocate for patients and biomedical research would support those experiments. Rather, the *language* in this exchange should attract our attention: It takes on a *scientistic* quality. Doerflinger grounds his concerns about a "class" of embryos in United States history and the decisions of the National Institutes of Health, while Perry depicts the progress of scientific experiments and uses that as a warrant for making a moral argument (*The NewsHour with Jim Lehrer,* 2000).

These language choices are not idiosyncratic to this one exchange and require further examination. While the different policy proposals, ethical stances, and political issues at play have been discussed in popular press books as well as academic work on ethics and politics (Cohen, 2007; Fox, 2007; Herold, 2006; Holland, Lebacqz, & Zoloth, 2001; Institute of Medicine, 2002), an examination of the public discourse on this issue and how the various strategies of definition and argument shape public attitudes toward stem cell research is missing. Almost all public debate about stem cells from 1998 through 2001 used language similar to that employed by Doerflinger and Perry in the PBS debate. Whereas topics of medical innovation and progress, the rights of fetuses, and the rights of patients make up the content addressed, each side is working hard to define what stem cells are in relation to those issues while doing so in language borrowed from science and scientific authorities. While each side of the debate is grounded in different social and political locations and while they view the issue through different cultural lenses, both sides turn to a *scientistic idiom,* a combination of scientific and quasi-scientific rhetorical strategies and key words. Individuals use this language to define what counts as real and thus embed their own values and ideological positions into the taken-for-granted assumptions that shape a debate. This book will examine the first stage of debate about ES cells from 1998 to 2001 and show how the debate focuses on arguments by definition that are developed in a science-like idiom of public argument. While the debate about ES cell research has continued since 2001, the vocabulary and strategies used to define ES cells were well established by the time President George W. Bush spoke on the issue in late 2001. Arguments since then have sometimes used combative or moralistic language that creates a Manichean framework in which the virtuous must defeat scientific attempts to re-create the world in the image of *Brave New World* or in which noble scientists must persevere in the face of religious persecution. Yet, the key issues are still those established prior to August 2001. Finally, a scientistic idiom was reasserted when President Barack Obama undid President Bush's restrictions on ES cell research in a speech on March 9, 2009. In order to understand the debate that continues to unfold, it is necessary to look back to when the definitions at the heart of the debate were fashioned, to identify the resources for rhetorical invention that were used, to see how they were mobilized, and to learn how they created our understanding of "stem cell" today.

Scientistic Idiom and Definition

Rhetors in the stem cell debate address three questions. First, why study ES cells? Scientists and politicians must define what ES cells are in a way that makes their study valuable. Second, are ES cells like fetuses? If they are, ES cell research violates the 1995 Dickey Amendment that forbids the destruction of human embryos in scientific research. Third, what is the relationship between embryonic and adult stem cells? If ES cells and adult stem cells are similar—if they have equivalent potencies or capabilities—then scientists and society have an alternative focus for research that does not raise moral objections about the life of the fetus. Answers to these three questions involve attempts at definition that cluster around the fundamental issue, "What are stem cells?" Furthermore, the answers to these questions express a variation of the public vernacular that I call "scientistic," or science-like.

Science-like idioms have appeared because science plays an increasing role in public deliberation (Beck, 1992; Irwin, 2001; Mitchell, 2000; Weingart, 2002). For some, this development represents the colonization of a weakened public sphere by the technical sphere and technoscientific modes of argument (Farrell & Goodnight, 1981; Goodnight, 1982; Irwin, 2001; Keränen, 2005). Others have noted that the application of scientific principles and practices to the public sphere undermines scientific claims to be the sole, objective source of information (Beck, 1992; Weingart, 2002). Finally, some claim that the movement of scientific issues into public forums highlights the interdependence and mutual influence science and the public have on each other (Boyd, 2002; Fabj & Sobnosky, 1995; Phillips, 1996; Taylor, 1996). Despite the variable judgments about the relative power science has over the public, these studies confirm John Lyne's observation that "the general culture incorporates scientific and quasi-scientific language, authority and modes of explanation into its talk about matters of common interest" (Lyne, 1996, p. 128).

Scholars have identified scientific and quasi-scientific modes of language used in multiple forums, but beyond the recognition of the link between science and popularized science, they do not consider how the language used moves beyond "common interest" to motivate collective action. Science journalism often appeals to potential applications and the experience of wonder in the face of nature's grandeur (Fahnestock, 1993). Popularizations of science often present a Baconian vision of science, which focuses on the object of investigation and portrays science as driven solely by empiricism and observation without theory (Curtis, 1994; Myers, 1990), and a host of different strategies have been used by scientists and lay audiences to render science intelligible (e.g., Fabj & Sobnosky, 1995; Fahnestock, 1999). Often, these modes of language appear in science-based controversies, and as Gordon Mitchell notes, "When truth claims packaged in the parlance of scientific objectivity meet resistance in deliberative forums, and open public debate ensues, the stage is set for public controversy. In this situation, argumentation can take a variety of forms and can occur in a multitude of different forums" (Mitchell, 2000, p. 17).

Yet, this variety of forms and forums is more than a corrupted derivation of scientific language; this variety does more than mimic science to create the illusion of understanding. Many of these rhetorical practices fulfill two functions for public deliberation. The first function is the creation of "real definitions," argumentative strategies establishing quasi-stable points from which individuals can make sense of the world and argue for various courses of action. The second function is to make these real definitions comport with the public's ideological commitments so they can become the basis for collective action. While this language, or vocabulary, exists on a continuum with science, the different goals and functions it fulfills distinguish it from a mere "quasi-scientific" language. I call it a *scientistic idiom* to recognize that the rhetorical strategies and arguments associated with science become a necessary component of public debate while those public debates become independent of the judgment of science and the technical sphere itself. In other words, the public sphere borrows scientific language while eschewing the scientific imprimatur for the use of that language.

Definition

Definitions are more than mere referential resources found in a dictionary and more than stipulations or temporary conveniences for the sake of exposition. Definition is a key step in any debate or discussion. As Zarefsky, Miller-Tutzauer, and Tutzauer (1984) note, "to choose a definition is to plead a cause . . . to name an object or idea is to influence attitudes about it" (p. 113). Furthermore, these definitions are themselves arguments (Perelman & Olbrechts-Tyteca, 1969, p. 213). As arguments, definitions appear in three modes: argument *from* definition, argument *about* definition, and argument *by* definition. Richard Weaver (1952) proposed the concept of argument *from* definition, where the definition acts like the major premise of a deductive argument; once one accepts the definition, the conclusions one draws about action and attitude are inevitable. Edward Schiappa (1993) discusses how many debates around definition are arguments *about* definition—debates concerning the appropriateness of a definition for a given case—instead of arguments from them, and David Zarefsky (1998) introduced the concept of argument *by* definition where the definition of a word, concept, or fragment is simply asserted during the course of argument.

According to Weaver, arguments from definition presuppose a belief that definitions are grounded in timeless or eternal essences: Arguments from definition aim at "getting people to see what is most permanent in existence, or what transcends the world of change and accident. The realm of essence is the realm above the flux of phenomena, and definitions are of essences and genres" (Weaver, 1952, p. 212). Chaim Perelman and Lucie Olbrechts-Tyteca (1969) identified dissociation as a strategy of definition, a strategy that prototypically divides a concept into its "appearance" and its "reality." Later scholarship on definition has emphasized that dissociation is the key strategy used by rhetors to create "real definitions" that determine what a concept "really" is (Goodwin, 1991; McGee, 1999; Schiappa, 1993, 2003). Contemporary scholars of communication and rhetoric have argued that practices of real definition typically involve dissociation and argument from definition, and they have argued that real definitions are products of naïve realism and a "picture theory" of language that ultimately treat definition as the identification of an absolute essence independent of human action and language use (Doyle, 1997; Goodwin, 1991; McGee, 1999; Schiappa, 1985, 1993, 1996, 2003; Titsworth, 1999; Walton, 2001).

This argument against real definitions and the rhetorical practices that make them possible is overextended in two ways. Some argue that creating definitions is conceptually impossible (Doyle, 1997). Others claim that certain forms of definition are irreparably tainted by naïve realism (Schiappa, 2003). These positions recognize the limitations of naïve realism, but they fail to account for how people define things and argue *by, from,* and *about* definition.[1] Definitions play a central role in many debates in science and in politics, but naïve realism is not the only perspective through which scholars can understand argument or the only way that publics approach definition. Definitions can change and develop over the course of a debate, which means they are not the identification of an "essence" or "reality" independent of the arguers or context of the debate. Instead, they provide a quasi-stable point from which individuals can make sense of the world and argue for various courses of action. Judgment calls about reality versus appearance occur every day in public rhetoric. Any individual arguing in the public sphere would be hard-pressed to avoid claims that some issues or objects are mere appearance belying the reality they perceive or experience.

Instead of eliminating real definitions or offering innumerable warnings about the contingent nature of our definitions, which is the antidote usually offered for definition's supposed essentialism (McGee, 1999; Schiappa, 2003), rhetorical scholars should reconfigure their understanding of real definitions and view them not as manifestations of a naïve realism but as the precondition for collective social action. Definitions play an important role in shaping people's psychosocial consensus about the world. This consensus determines what counts as "real" for a given group of people. The "real" underlying collective action is not the "reality" of naïve realism: We should understand "the real" as a psychosocial consensus about the world and naïve realism's "reality" as a construct stipulating the independence of the world from our perception (Goodwin, 1991; Lynch, 2006). This means that what counts as "real" will both change depending on the groups engaged in definition and evolve over time. Proponents and opponents in the debate about ES cell research offer various definitions of "stem cell" in scientific, political, and journalistic forums. While these definitions will have similarities, this is a result of similar issues playing across different contexts. As those issues change and diversify—for example, when scientists debate a specific finding, or politicians consider the minutiae of funding decisions, or journalists shift from discussing stem cells as a political issue toward discussing it as an issue for business and investment—the specific arguments from, about, and by definition will change.

Definition's capacity for creating our consensus about the "real" dovetails with the positioning of science as the source of objective knowledge about the world, and it is also reinforced by the practice of argument *by* definition. The arguments made through definition can become the basis for collective action more readily when the definition is treated as a matter-of-fact observation the arguer merely notes in passing. By treating a definition as a fact and presenting it in language borrowed from science, one bolsters the strength of the argument by making it appear as a feature of the world beyond debate. The more prosaic and noncontroversial a definition appears, the better it fulfills its function. Yet, argument by definition will not always be possible. Sometimes an arguer will be forced to show his or her hand and argue from definition in order to make the implications for action clear, but this opens up the possibility for later argument *about* that definition.

Link to American Ideology

In addition to providing real definitions, scientistic idioms must offer definitions that comport with American ideological commitments. While ideology has a broad range of meanings and uses (Eagleton, 1991, pp. 1–31; Williams, 1983, pp. 153–157), I follow Robert Asen and understand ideology as "a strategic set of claims, values and beliefs that advocates may invoke to build collectives, forge alliances, and highlight differences," as well as shaping our consensus about the taken-for-granted facts about a given issue (Asen, 2009, p. 266). The link to ideology does not mean that scientistic idioms are reducible to biorhetoric, where individuals transform moral statements into naturalistic or factual statements (Lyne, 1990). Instead, scientistic idioms use real definitions to provide "facts" that shape a debate and become the fodder for ethical and moral judgment. As Ulrich Beck (1992) notes in his discussion of risk and science, "'facts'—the former centerpieces of reality—are nothing but answers to questions that could just as well have been asked differently, products of rules for gathering and omitting" (p. 166).[2] All parties in a debate will try to provide facts and evidence to support their moral judgment, and they will try to present those facts as agreed-upon statements derived from a scientific consensus (see Weingart, 2002). While argument by definition is the primary strategy for establishing what counts as real in a given debate, the definitions offered must comport themselves with American ideological commitments in order to motivate collective action. Such an explicit connection to ideology would seem to undermine the *appearance* of scientific objectivity, but four factors mitigate this.

First, a scientistic idiom, like most scientific rhetoric, avoids explicit value statements, thus forcing opponents of any specific use of this vocabulary to impute that bias exists and convince others to see that bias as well. This, in part, helps explain Schiappa's observation that most attempts at arguing from definition rapidly devolve into arguments *about* definition: The stakes are too high to allow any attempt at definition to go unchallenged (Schiappa, 1993). Second, the acceptance of any given definition as real, especially when it can be supported by scientific or quasi-scientific observations about a phenomenon, undermines the ability to attack the definition as ideological or partisan: A definition's role in determining the consensus about the real makes unpacking its ideological components difficult, but not impossible. Definitions can change or be supplanted, and those changes often involve revealing the ideological underpinning of any given definition to invalidate its claim to be "real." Third, when contrasted with explicitly political rhetoric that appears in campaigns and explicitly religious rhetoric, science usually appears less biased. American tradition and the First Amendment call for separation of church and state, and they have portrayed political and religious rhetoric as having an inherent bias. Given such obvious examples of ideological bias to provide a foil, other rhetorics and vocabularies will find it easier to avoid such labels.

Fourth, unlike political and religious rhetorics, a scientistic idiom can be used by anyone regardless of his or her politics or religion. While the idiom requires speakers to avoid explicit value statements, some religious and political arguments can be deployed in a scientistic idiom. It is often valuable for religious and political individuals to use that language because it acts as "an implicit, objectivized manipulation of latently political variables" (Beck, 1992, p. 170). To the extent that groups are adept at adjusting to this language, they can incorporate their concerns into a given debate in ways that minimize the appearance of partisanship. This does not mean religious arguments cast in a scientistic idiom will necessarily succeed: "Different forms of expertise may not easily combine, as they may represent fundamentally different lifeworlds and ways of framing an issue" (Leach & Scoones, 2005, p. 18). Reframing religious or political concerns into a scientistic idiom can potentially be difficult and will not go unchallenged by opponents. Also, scientistic idioms will not always be the most effective means of persuasion and will not always win every science-based controversy; while they have a natural advantage when it comes to arguing about what counts as "real" and shaping a consensus on collective action, religious and political vocabularies will be available as well and might still be in play in these debates. I argue here that the stem cell debate occurs primarily in a scientistic idiom, but other science-based controversies will have other languages play a major, or dominant, role. Evolution is one situation where the debate is primarily framed around religious objections to a scientific theory.[3] Religious sentiments and vocabulary have the upper hand in that debate in America. Also, even in cases where a scientistic idiom dominates the debate, the arguments about and by definition will be heated and long running: Success will be partial and elusive.

Real definitions must align with American ideological commitments in order to motivate people to support a collective action, such as funding ES cell research. Unlike the public consultation efforts common in Europe (Joss & Durant, 1995; Leach & Scoones, 2005), scientistic idioms are not informational campaigns. Rather, they are the mode of public discourse through which a general public engages science and science-based controversies. Scientistic idioms make science useful and meaningful for a deliberating public. This results in an idiom that is always contingent and partial. It is contingent because the specific elements of the idiom will reflect the scientific findings at hand and the specific issues related to those findings that are politically and culturally salient. It is partial because it represents only one of the socioeconomic, cultural, and rhetorical forces that can shape science-based controversies. This means the scope of a scientistic idiom cannot be fully determined: The substance of real definitions and the other strategies extant within a scientistic idiom draw on an open-ended set of rhetorical figures and arguments, thus producing the multitude of strategies and arguments noted by others. While the scope of possible figures and arguments is theoretically broad, specific debates will coalesce around a set of key strategies as individuals identify the contours of that debate and the issues on which they can shift the public consensus.

Delineating Science, Scientism, and Scientistic Idioms

I have defined a scientistic idiom as a set of rhetorical figures and arguments organized around the goal of defining what counts as "real" in a given debate and insuring that reality comports with the public's ideological commitments, but the differences between science and scientistic vocabularies on the one hand, and scientistic vocabularies and an ideology of scientism, on the other, require further clarification. This is partly due to the amorphous boundary between science and nonscience (Boyd, 2002; Gieryn, 1983; Keränen, 2005; Lessl, 1988; Taylor, 1996). Also, there is a necessary degree of overlap between all three concepts. Scientistic idioms and scientism would not exist if not for the modern practice of science.

Science

While the boundaries between science broadly construed and nonscientific activities are fluid, we can identify some basic qualities of science. Science is the practice of establishing "facts." Ideally, this occurs through the generation and testing of hypotheses, although science studies have shown how science repeatedly falls short of this ideal (e.g., Collins, 1992; Nelson, Megill, & McCloskey, 1987; Pickering, 1984; Simons, 1990). Scientific practice welds together things and symbols into the fusion of "facts" that society treats as having greater epistemic purchase than the observations produced in nonscientific practices (Latour, 1987; Lynch, 2009; Shapin & Schaffer, 1985). Scientific practice usually occurs in laboratories, although field observations, ice core sampling, and other activities occurring outside of a lab are also part of the scientific creation of facts. While the term is traditionally associated with the spaces where biology, chemistry, and physics occur, laboratories can also be other physical spaces like factories and virtual spaces like computer networks (Miller & Oleary, 1994; Mody, 2005).

This definition of science is broad for two reasons. First, the demarcation of science from nonscience is symbolically and rhetorically mediated: While people have a broad sense of what is "scientific," the specific practices labeled "science" are contingent and change with historical and social developments (Gieryn, 1983; Taylor, 1996). For example, 19th-century science was demarcated to exclude both religious authority and the work of engineers who invented machines like the steam engine (Gieryn, 1983). Second, the range of "science" is expanding, as the practices defined as "scientific" in the contemporary era are brought to bear on new areas of the world and human life (Boyd, 2002; Keränen, 2005; Latour, 1987). For example, the discourse and practices of psychiatry have become a common thread in the fabric of everyday life (Johnson, 2008; Rodriguez, 2006). In order to have a definition of science that is not bound to one historical moment, one must have a theoretically broad definition able to reflect and respond to the shifting historical nature of science: Rhetorical criticism of science must then be theoretically broad in defining its object even as it becomes critically narrowed in selecting a specific time period and the practices demarcated as "scientific" at that time.

Scientism and Manichean Idioms

Scientism is an ideology that aggrandizes science and its epistemic power (Lessl, 2007; McCloskey, 1998).[4] It consists of "the tendency to enlarge beyond warrant the cognitive bounds of science" (Lessl, 1996, p. 379). It also has a tendency to collapse other forms of knowledge into scientific ones, claiming, like E. O. Wilson did, that moral or artistic sentiments are determined by nature or biology (Ceccarelli, 2001, chapter 6; Lessl, 1996). In its creation of a dichotomy between scientific knowledge and other epistemic regimes, scientism embodies a Manichean idiom. Manichean idioms create the appearance of two opposing sides where there is no room for compromise. Rhetoricians of science have often focused on pro-science Manichean idioms, as embodied by studies of scientism, but pro-religion or pro-society versions are also possible (Lessl, 1999, 2002, 2007; Johnson, 2006). Pro-religion versions of the idiom share the focus on creating a dichotomy with no room for compromise, but here the role is to obstruct scientific practice and act as an "epistemological filibuster" (Paroske, 2009). Often, arguments in this idiom will draw on the figure of Frankenstein's monster or the book *Brave New World* as a source of rhetorical invention, as will be shown in detail later.

Some have argued that presenting scientific debates increases public engagement (Mooney & Nisbet, 2005). Scholars studying mass media and science journalism have argued that conflict provides the space for providing more information through media channels as well as increasing the public's knowledge and engagement with an issue (Nisbet & Goidel, 2007; Nisbet & Huge, 2006; Olien, Donohue, & Tichenor, 1995; Wilcox, 2003). This capacity of conflict to foster engagement and increase knowledge has limits. As Olien, Donohue, and Tichenor (1995) note, "while conflict situations often stimulate communication, interest and thought, a point of public disinterest and even disgust may be reached in conflicts that are perceived to be without resolution" (p. 317). Manichean idioms, whether supportive of science or opposed to it, diminish the positive impact of conflict because they present an issue as having no possible compromises. With the possibility of a policy acceptable to all sides eliminated a priori, the value of conflict is eliminated, leaving only the possibility of acrimony.

The Scientistic Idiom

In contrast to science and scientism, a scientistic idiom articulates a relationship between science and the public that enables collective public action based on what is perceived as "real." Science exists as a set of practices that examine the world and those within it, but the relationship between science, politics, and other realms of human experience is shifting and often tumultuous. Scientistic idioms work to manage that relationship. Scientism represents an ideology that argues for the supremacy of science and scientific findings. Scientistic idioms borrow from the language of science, but they do not require those who use them to adhere to every scientific qualification and quibble, which the ideology of scientism would demand. Society has "become more dependent on scientific arguments *in general,* but at the same time more independent of *individual* findings and the judgment of science regarding the truth and reality of its statements" (Beck, 1992, p. 167). While arguments will take on the appearance of science and use some of its rhetorical strategies, collective public action does not depend on scientific approval and can actively disregard science if it runs counter to public desires or values. This occurs for two reasons. First, science has grown so large and so specialized that nonscientists trying to understand science must judge it using their own criteria: "The flood of findings, their contradictoriness and overspecialization, turn reception into participation, into an autonomous process of knowledge formation *with and against* science" (Beck, 1992, p. 167). Second, scientific expertise is available to all sides in a debate, thus allowing proponents and opponents of an issue or initiative to present "scientific" evidence that supports opposing points of view (Weingart, 2002).

Scientistic idioms have an element of translation, but a scientistic idiom should not be reduced to the translation of a concept. Concepts and concerns move between the science and the public. Rhetoricians, sociologists, and social psychologists have developed a number of broad models to describe the movement, alternately described as "translation" or "popularization," of ideas and technology from the laboratory to the public (Fabj & Sobnosky, 1995; Latour, 1987; Latour & Woolgar, 1986; Moscovici, 1984; Wagner & Kronberger, 2001). But, these models of translation are limited for two reasons. First, as Massimiano Bucchi (1998) notes, the process of translation is often viewed as unidirectional and discrete: Scientists or their intermediaries explain science to a public after the scientific findings have already been finalized. This viewpoint does not consider how scientists translate concepts from the popular culture when they begin the process of defining scientific concepts and objects. Second, these models— especially Latour's model (1987)—have been criticized as mechanistic or "brute force" models that allow the scientist with the greatest number of facts and most expensive "toys" or experimental apparatus to win (Gross, 1990). More nuanced perspectives, like those found in the work of Beck (1992) and Weingart (2002), also fail to account for the role of persuasion, instead focusing on structural issues like the economic power, access to media, and access to experts one can hire to support one's views. The role of the rhetorical—the element of the broader cultural sphere involved with the configuration of discourse and argument—is downplayed in these accounts.

Overview

In many arguments, defining is half the battle. Those who successfully define an object, idea, or group make the process of persuading their audience easier, and make the task of their opposition more difficult. Definition has become the central strategy in scientistic idioms that work to establish what counts as real for debates about public action and policy and make that sense of the real consonant with American ideological commitments. Rhetors in the ES cell debate try to portray themselves and their concerns within a scientistic idiom, rather than a religious or partisan idiom, while using various strategies to define ES cells to their advantage.

Three strategies played key roles in the definition of stem cells: appeals to application or ends, appeals to source or origin, and what I will call the argument from hierarchy. These strategies were used by multiple rhetors to create definitions of "stem cell" and "embryonic stem cell" in order to shift the grounds for debating the merits of federal funding for this research. There is no a priori ordering or logic of these three strategies. In principle, the combination of these three strategies can lead to a number of positions: For example, some people affiliated with the right-to-life movement recognize the possible medical benefit of ES cell research but oppose it because ES cells are derived from embryos, while some feminists like Judy Norsigian of the Boston Women's Health Book Collective object to ES cell research *not* because they have explicit concerns about the embryo, but because acquiring embryos from which to derive ES cells can adversely affect women's health; and they feel adult stem cells are as powerful as ES cells. Yet some combinations of these strategies have greater traction in the public sphere, and the debates during this early stage of the stem cell controversy became deadlocked: Concerns about the embryo were balanced against the value of possible medical applications. Neither side gained sufficient political and social capital to force the issue in their favor. While arguments about the equivalent potency of adult stem cells were dealt a blow by scientific findings in early 2002, the political argument remained deadlocked with George W. Bush's policy on ES cell research. Bush's speech announced his decision to fund research only on ES cell lines derived before August 9, 2001, and his decision reflected the tensions within the political debate. His speech used a Manichean idiom with religion and morality opposing the potential for scientific excess and overreach, and it combined the prevalent definitions in this debate—ES cells destroyed human life *and* could potentially save human life. Public discourse about ES cells following Bush's speech remained in a stalemate, until President Barack Obama's speech in 2009 announced the lifting of the Bush restrictions on ES cell research and returned the discussion of ES cells to a scientistic idiom. This book analyzes attempts to define "stem cell" within a scientistic idiom and how those attempts at scientistic definition have been shadowed by a Manichean idiom contrasting the forces of good (typically, religion or morality) and evil (typically science).[5]

Chapter 2 addresses the ends of research—specific applications scientists and politicians hope that ES cell research will yield. Application—the "why" for stem cell research—plays a key role in both scientific and political rhetoric since it can be linked to ideas of the common good and to care for others as well as a pragmatic, technologically oriented mindset (in other words, the desire for technological fixes for a problem instead of political or behavioral changes). Yet, these applications exist in a possible future, so the issue of timing, or *kairos,* becomes a key part of the definition. ES cells and research on them are defined as the best—the timeliest—way to achieve the applications desired by scientists and the public. In science, three applications appear: stem cells can help increase understandings of basic biology, stem cells can be used for screening new pharmaceuticals, and stem cells can be used to cure diseases for which no cure currently exists, such as Parkinson's disease and diabetes. In political discourse, all three of the applications appear, but medical applications—the use of stem cells for curing disease—take the fore because they generate the most appeal for lay audiences. The emphasis on different potential applications changes the biological qualities considered key to defining "stem cell." Yet, these applications are only *potential* applications, and it is their potentiality—the uncertainty about whether or not present research will yield future application—that plays a major role in political definition by application. Proponents of this research must shape the definition by application so that stem cells, especially ES cells, represent the quickest path to the largest number of potential applications, while opponents of ES cell research emphasize the uncertainty inherent in deliberative discourse about future applications.

The origin of ES cells in 15-day-old embryos becomes the crux of many arguments opposing ES cell research, and definitions associating and dissociating ES cells and embryos are the focus of chapters 3 and 4. These arguments are grounded in the same concern for others that motivates the call for medical applications, although embryos are the focus of concern here, as well as religious objections to interfering with the beginnings of human life. Chapter 3 addresses the initial attempts by journalists to frame this issue and by opponents to use resources from the abortion debate to define ES cells. Journalists use contemporary debates about abortion to frame the ES cell debate and explain opposition to this research, and they often frame the debate as one of religious opposition to scientific research. Yet, journalists must also account for the fact that some prominent pro-life politicians support ES cell research. Many opponents of ES cell research turn to the rhetorical image of the "public fetus" common in right-to-life arguments to define ES cells as embryos or inextricably link them to the destruction of embryonic life, but some of them, especially politicians in the House and Senate, explicitly disavow connections between the abortion debate and the ES cell debate. This situation highlights the challenge of translating objections to ES cell research grounded in religious public vocabularies associated with the right-to-life movement into a scientistic public vocabulary. Journalists and politicians each use a variety of different strategies to explain this situation and make their definitions effective.

Proponents of ES cell research do not leave these challenges unanswered. Chapter 4 discusses the two primary strategies of proponents, as well as attempts by opponents to reply to these counters. Proponents define "spare embryos" as those embryos that have no chance of developing into human beings and that offer a viable source for stem cells, and some proponents also try to define the earliest stages of human life as "pre-embryos" that have a different moral value than born humans and fetuses at later stages of development. In all of these definitions and counter-definitions about origin, there is a tendency to move beyond a scientistic idiom and engage in biorhetoric, the transformation of moral judgments into natural "fact" (Lyne, 1990). These chapters map out this tension between a scientistic idiom and biorhetoric, and they highlight the dangers in attempts to camouflage ethical thinking as a discovered quality of biology.

Chapter 5 addresses how categories of stem cells are defined and organized in relation to each other. The argument from hierarchy is used to create a ranking of stem cell types based on different "potencies," or the capacity of stem cells to produce different types of cells. The hierarchy defines ES cells as more powerful than adult stem cells: ES cells have pluripotency, compared to the multipotency of adult stem cells. Yet, the argument from hierarchy contains ambiguities that can be deployed to trouble the rankings of the two categories of stem cells. Ideologically, this argument reflects the human condition of being "goaded by hierarchy"—and thus fulfills a universal human tendency or need—but it also reflects the pragmatic focus of debates on ES cell research (Burke, 1966, pp. 15–16). Arguments from hierarchy also highlight the interplay of science and the scientistic idiom. Both scientific and public discourses use the same hierarchy to construct arguments and organize cell types. Yet scientific and public discourses produce different types of claims, and scientists speaking in the public sphere cannot disbar or refute public claims contrary to their own.

Chapter 6 addresses presidential rhetoric about stem cells, specifically President Bush's first televised address on August 9, 2001, announcing limited support for ES cell research and President Obama's speech overturning that decision. President Bush's speech builds on the definitions of ES cell developed in a scientistic idiom, but he recasts the issue in a Manichean language in which science and morality struggle against each other. This produces an incoherent definition—ES cells simultaneously destroy and save lives—which renders the policy he announces incoherent. Despite this, his policy stands, and his Manichean framing of the issue resonates in public discourse over the next seven years. Then, with President Obama's announcement lifting the Bush-era restrictions on ES cell research, there is a return to a scientistic idiom and an attempt to inoculate public discourse against further attempts at Manichean definition of science and ES cell research.

2

Timely and Powerful

Defining Stem Cells through Appeals to Application

The applications of scientific research—how the results of research can be used to further a scientific or societal purpose—are possibilities, nothing more than a hypothetical conjecture, but "the determination and operationalization of consequences, hypothetical conjectures and the like are therefore levers with which fundamental decisions on the social future are carried out" (Beck, 1992, p. 174). Scientists and nonscientists both ask, "Why study stem cells?" The answer usually refers back to some larger project whether it is epistemic, pecuniary, or humanitarian. Another way to think about potential applications is to think about the opportunities presented by stem cell research. Rhetoricians from ancient Greece to modern times have recognized the creation or the perception of opportunity as *kairos,* the "right time" or opportune moment for using words to create an advantage for oneself. *Kairos* and the appeal to application become central strategies for defining stem cells in a scientistic idiom. Furthermore, *kairos* and the appeal to application appear in both scientific and public rhetoric, highlighting the translation of concepts across the public and technical spheres. How the opportunities from this research are presented shapes the definition of stem cells as well as the sense of urgency around federal funding for this research. Yet the presentation of opportunity, the promise of future applications, opens up the grounds for arguments from opposing rhetors.

Kairos, Opportunity, and Application

For the ancient Greeks, *kairos* meant many things: It referred to timing, but it also meant symmetry, propriety, profit, fitness, opening, and the fatal spot targeted by archers (Hawhee, 2004; Miller, 1992; Sipiora, 2002; J. E. Smith, 2002). *Kairos* as it relates to speech highlights a qualitative character of time, in contrast to the sense of time as a quantitative measure (J. E. Smith, 2002). Carolyn Miller argues that temporal and spatial understandings of *kairos* are key to persuasion:

Not only must the individual speak or write at the proper time, he or she must also find the right "opening," the right point of entry into a subject or an ongoing debate, if he or she wishes to be successful (Miller, 1992).

Both classical and modern understandings of *kairos* recognize a tension between the objective and subjective (Hawhee, 2004; Miller, 1994; Scott, 2006). Debate continues about how to theorize the indeterminacy of *kairos,* specifically whether thinking about *kairos* must go beyond the recognition of an uncertain future and highlight the risks of the undesired effects of acting and speaking in the present (Scott, 2006). Miller, though, provides a way of resolving these issues in the context of science and technology. She argues for viewing *kairos* as the interplay of objective and subjective forces in any situation: Any speaker or writer takes the facts of the situation as they exist and recasts them to create a sense of urgency and opportunity (Miller, 1992, 1994). In a sense, a rhetor redefines the situation so that it becomes an urgent moment to seize an opportunity. In the case of stem cell research, the existence of adult and embryonic stem cells is the objective condition necessary for individual scientists and politicians to argue that timely financial support is needed. Given this, individuals have a great deal of power to recast the situation of ES cell research in words and symbols to create a sense of urgency and opportunity. Yet, because *kairos* projects a path from an indeterminate present into an uncertain future, the possibility of failure and risk "is always inherent in *kairos*" (Scott, 2006, p. 119).

Creating a timely opening or opportunity for present action to lead to a projected (hoped-for) future occurs in both scientific rhetoric and the scientistic idiom. In both cases, the opportunity is understood as future applications: Scientific and policy debates about potential technologies create "opportunities for opportunity" (Miller, 1994, p. 93)—opening the space for a project to move from concept to execution—and the appeal to applications has been recognized as a key component of media presentations of science and technology (Fahnestock, 1993).[1] Appeals to application drive the stem cell debate by defining stem cells as an opportunity for creating a better future. Thus, the use of definition creates a sense of a "real" opportunity to achieve the ends of science and society. Yet, the specifics of this *kairos* change between the scientific and political arenas. The discourse of science uses three broad appeals: an appeal to research, an appeal to pharmaceutical screening, and an appeal to regenerative medicine. The political discourse primarily focuses on one appeal: an appeal to regenerative medicine. This shift in applications helps illustrate how the *kairos* of stem cell research is a blending of objective and subjective elements. When individuals shift the range of appeals they use, the qualities of stem cells that are important for realizing this future shift as well. Also, fundamental uncertainty about the future forces individuals advocating for stem cell research in the political arena to amplify the scope of application and claim that the promise of stem cell research will be realized in the near future, thus exposing them to the risk of promising too much and also creating the opportunity for opponents of the research to challenge the promise of research and the act of making that promise.

Scientific Appeals to Application

In scientific rhetoric about stem cells, there are three broad applications explicitly discussed: using stem cells to gain an understanding of the earliest events in mammalian, especially human, development; using stem cells to create "screens," or specialized cell samples, to use in testing new drugs; and using stem cells to create replacements for tissues destroyed by many diseases and degenerative conditions. These applications would fill gaps in existing biomedical knowledge and practices, but the possibility of realizing these applications exists in a far-flung future. *Kairos* lies in making other scientists feel that believing in this work and developing their own projects in the area of stem cell research will position them to profit, financially and intellectually, from future applications. With the exception of scientific articles published before the isolation of human ES cells (Evans & Kaufman, 1981; Gardner & Beddington, 1988; Martin, 1981; Thomson et al., 1995) and review articles specifically addressing how to translate this research into medical settings (e.g. Weissman, 2000b), most articles address the full range of applications. Thomson et al. (1998) note, "These cell lines should be useful in human developmental biology, drug discovery, and transplantation medicine" (p. 1145). Shamblott et al. (1998) claim stem cells "would be invaluable for studies of some aspects of human embryogenesis and for transplantation therapies" (p. 13730). Watt and Hogan (2000) claim studies of stem cells "hold great promise not only for unexpected insights into biology but ultimately for the alleviation of human suffering" (p. 1430). While discussion of application usually focuses on ES cells, some research articles on adult stem cells discuss possible applications as well. For example, Jackson, Mi, and Goodell (1999) claim, "If stem cells from adult tissues are generally found to have a broad potential to differentiate, it may not be necessary to use embryonic stem cells in some medical and experimental settings" (p. 14485).

The most detailed list of applications comes from Austin Smith (2001), whose discussion of future applications also highlights the qualities of ES cells necessary to achieve these ends:

> The dual capacities of mouse ES cells for unlimited expansion and for multilineage differentiation have subsequently provoked interest in estab-

lishing similar embryo-derived cell lines of human origin. The motivations for this are essentially fourfold:

a. human embryology—to recapitulate in vitro otherwise inaccessible aspects of early differentiation of the human embryo;
b. functional genomics—to investigate and manipulate specific gene functions in diploid human cells;
c. pharmaceutical development—to provide large numbers of phenotypically defined human cell types for compound screening and toxicological testing;
d. regenerative medicine—to create a renewable supply of cells for clinical use in cell replacement, tissue repair and delivery of gene therapy. (p. 449–450)

Smith creates a fourfold sense of *kairotic* opportunity: This present work on ES cells creates the opportunity for better understanding of human development and genetics, testing new pharmaceuticals, and creating the field of regenerative medicine. This future depends on two "objective" or situational factors. First, current biomedical practices lack tools to address the areas Smith identifies. Second, two qualities found in present-day stem cells can be redefined as the means to achieve these ends: the capacity to expand the population of stem cells for an unlimited period (also known as self-renewal) and the capacity to differentiate (to become many different types of specialized cells).

In the core set of 50 scientific research and review articles on stem cells that are cited the most frequently from 1998 to 2001, both concepts are mentioned with a similar frequency: "self-renewal" appears 31 times, while "differentiation" appears 40 times.[2] The difference is attributable to the brief reports on adult stem cells that focus on their capacity to differentiate. These two characteristics become the *defining* characteristics of stem cells, especially ES cells. Thomson and Odorico (2000) begin their review of ES cell research with this definitional move: "The essential characteristics of all stem cells are prolonged self-renewal and the long-term potential to form one or more differentiated cell types" (p. 53). Slack (2000) notes, "A consensus definition is likely to include at least two ideas: stem cells are able to reproduce themselves throughout the lifespan of the animal, and they are able to give rise to differentiated cells" (p. 1431). Weissman (2000a) says, "Stem cells are generally defined as clonogenic cells capable of both self-renewal and multilineage differentiation" (p. 157). In each of these cases, stem cells are defined as cells that have a capacity for self-renewal and a capacity for differentiation, and the existence of these capacities in the present creates the possibility for future applications. While these statements present these qualities as a matter of fact, their location in the introduction of each article also means they act like an argument from definition. As in the example from Smith quoted above, the future applications are deduced from the present qualities of the cells.

Scientists present stem cell research as the key to several potential applications in research, drug discovery, and transplantation medicine. Most often, these appeals to application in scientific literature are associated with ES cells, but occasionally scientists mention the application of adult stem cells. Discussion of stem cells is organized around *kairos,* the creation of future opportunity. This opportunity is grounded in the selection of key attributes already identified in stem cells, but it also functions because of the lack of knowledge about stem cells. Many details about ES cells and their capacity to differentiate (especially the ability to control that process) were, and still are, unclear; this provides scientific rhetors a "blank canvas" on which to paint their picture of the future. *Kairos* also plays a role in popular rhetoric about stem cells, but the future opportunities and applications become narrowed in these areas to emphasize medical application.

Appeals to Medical Application in Politics and Journalism

Like scientific discourse, political appeals to future applications focus on ES cells, but the exact form they take changes in the move from scientific to popular discussion. Popular discussions of stem cell research focus on the possible medical applications of stem cells more than the research and pharmaceutical applications. In the congressional hearings on stem cell research from 1998 to 2001, all three applications are mentioned together in 14 individual testimonies, but medical applications appear alone in over 60 testimonies. Application to basic research appears alone in 10 testimonies, and pharmaceutical applications appear alone in only one testimony. In the 303 news stories sampled, appeals to medical applications appear in 212 stories. Research and pharmaceutical applications appear in 20 and 7 stories, respectively, and they always appear as secondary applications.

The range of applications narrows because the role of the audience in the present moment changes. In scientific discourse, part of the purpose is to recruit other scientists into stem cell research: Present action will lead to future applications and future rewards for scientists who act on this promise. With popular discourse, support is reflected by a change of opinion in the general public and a support for funding on the part of politicians. The future depicted must be salient to nonscientific publics. The drive for basic knowledge does not have a broad appeal, and the degree of detail inherent in many basic biological questions makes it difficult to translate the appeal of basic research into a form larger audiences can appreciate. The creation of cell cultures to screen drugs does not appeal to a large nonscience audience because pharmaceutical companies, rather than people, are the primary beneficiaries of this application.[3]

Medical applications appeal directly to mass audiences because all individuals can benefit, in theory, from new medical discoveries. Any individual might succumb to Alzheimer's disease, Parkinson's disease, diabetes, heart attack, or stroke; therefore, any individual could potentially benefit from cures derived from ES cells. Even if a person avoids one of these conditions, he or she is likely to know at least one person who suffers or dies from one of them, and medical applications will impact their lives by providing cures or treatments for friends and family. Speakers in the political realm recognize the personal connection individuals can have to the medical applications of stem cell research. They can use the potential benefits to the lay public as a means of appealing to them. The medical applications of stem cell research become not only the "real definition" of stem cells but also the primary means of comporting this research and government support for it with American values.

Some scientists who speak in political forums try to deploy all three scientific appeals to application, but even then, the medical applications take priority. Sometimes, this priority manifests itself in the order in which the appeals are presented. For example, in his prepared statement for the first congressional hearing on stem cell research, Dr. James Thomson said,

> Human ES cell lines are important because they could provide large, purified populations of human cells such as heart muscle cells, pancreatic cells or neurons for transplantation therapies. . . . Human ES cells are also important because they will offer insights into the developmental events that cannot be studied directly in the intact human embryo, but which have important consequences in clinical areas, including birth defects, infertility, and pregnancy loss. Screening tests that use specific ES cell derivatives will allow the identification of new drugs, the identification of genes that could be used for tissue regeneration therapies, and the identification of toxic compounds. (*Stem Cell Research,* 1999, p. 16)

Although the wording of this section is almost identical to the list of applications from Thomson et al.'s article (1998) announcing the isolation of ES cells, the order in which they appear has changed. The structure of the testimony creates a temporal priority for medical application over the other two applications.

Additionally, testimony by scientists who address all three applications amplifies the importance of medical applications because of the quantity of testimony devoted to it. During the first hearing on stem cell research, National Institutes of Health (NIH) director Harold Varmus presents all three applications in the same order as they appear in scientific rhetoric—first, basic research; then, pharmaceutical applications; and finally, medical applications—but he devotes only one paragraph each to the first two applications and four to medical applications, providing extended examples about curing type I diabetes and repairing damaged heart tissue (*Stem Cell Research*, 1999, p. 9). He repeats this pattern almost two months later during the second round of hearings before the Senate Appropriations Subcommittee on Labor, Health and Human Services, and Education (*Stem Cell Research*, 1999, p. 122).

In contrast to the testimony of scientists during the first hearing on stem cell research, most popular discourse focused on medical applications alone, and following the first round of hearings, many scientists do the same thing. In a November 1999 hearing, Sen. Strom Thurmond (R-SC) remarks, "I am hopeful that we are on the verge of discovering a whole new way of treating and curing diseases which for too long have led to pain and suffering in the lives of too many Americans" (*Stem Cell Research, part 2,* 1999, p. 19). An early CNN news report on stem cells announces, "Researchers hope stem cells can be removed and customized to repair virtually any damaged human tissue" ("Presidential Ethics Panel," 1998). When research is mentioned, rhetors emphasize the contribution of basic research to understanding health and medical issues. For example, Sen. Tom Harkin (D-IA) opens two different rounds of testimony with the observation that ES cell research increases "our understanding of human development and cancer biology" (*Stem Cell Research,* 1999, p. 93). Observation of human development is linked with understanding cancer, which presumably would lead to cures. An article in the *Omaha World Herald* makes a similar observation about birth defects: ES cells "are the only window that researchers have to early human development, and Thomson said they could reveal ways to detect and remedy birth defects" (Olson, 2000e). Following the first round of testimony in 1998, many scientists began to address only medical applications. For example, in January 1999, Dr. Douglas Melton of Harvard discusses how ES cells could lead to a cure for type I diabetes, and Dr. Lawrence Goldstein notes that ES cells "have extraordinary potential to revolutionize the treatment and cure of devastating human diseases" (*Stem Cell Research,* 1999, p. 97).

Medical appeals are the primary focus of popular rhetoric about stem cells. Even when rhetors repeat the language of application found in scientific discourse, medical applications are foregrounded. In addition to this shift in the applications addressed, three things occur with popular appeals to medical applications. First, the change in the range of applications appealed to also changes the qualities of stem cells that make them important. Second, appeals to medical applications define ES cell research as the best and most advantageous route to medical therapies for currently incurable diseases. Third, rhetors who appeal to medical applications must respond to concerns about the timeliness of ES cell research and create a timeline for when medical applications will become widely available, thus defining ES cells as the *quickest* route to therapies. This timeline is ambiguous, and detailed questioning about it leads proponents of ES cell research to create multiple caveats displacing responsibility for meeting the goals identified in the timeline from scientists to the NIH bureaucracy or opponents of ES cell research.

The Timely Qualities of Stem Cells

Since *kairos* creates a trajectory from the indeterminate present to the hoped-for future, a shift in the future creates a shift in the qualities of the present that will lead to that future. With the narrowing of the range of future applications attributed to stem cell research, the qualities most salient to realizing that future narrow as well. In scientific discourse, the qualities of "self-renewal" and "differentiation" play equally important roles. In popular discourse, "differentiation" becomes the most important quality. Differentiation is the stem cell's capacity to become any type of cell, and this quality makes it ideal for regenerative medicine. This shift in emphasis to "differentiation" alone first becomes apparent with the number of times each quality is mentioned. "Self-renewal" appears 11 times in political discourse and 12 times in journalistic discourse, while "differentiation" appears 35 times in political discourse and 28 times in journalistic discourse. The emphasis on differentiation also appears explicitly. Dr. Douglas Melton, in his prepared statement for the Senate Appropriations Subcommittee, says, "Stem cells have the potential to develop into any tissue or organ in the body" (*Stem Cell Research,* 1999, p. 101). Melton's statement emphasizes the capacity for stem cells to differentiate, to become different types of cells and tissue.

The emphasis on differentiation over self-renewal also appears in the variety of ways that journalists translate these scientific terms into everyday language. Typically, journalists describe self-renewal as the capacity stem cells have for "dividing indefinitely" ("Embryonic Stem Cell Research," 2001; Mishra, 2001c; Stolberg, 2001c) and "living forever" (Hesman, 2000). Journalists say stem cells show "versatility" when describing differentiation (Friend, 2001c; Hesman, 2001b; Kiely, 2001a), or journalists describe stem cells' capacity for differentiation as the capacity to "grow" new tissues for the body (Abate, 2000; "Debate over Embryonic," 2001; "Scientists and Anti-Abortion," 2001; Ward, 2000; Weiss, 2000a; Zitner, 1999) or "transform" into different types of tissue ("Here's What Debate," 2001; Nelson, 2000; Pollack, 2001a; "President Bush to Announce," 2001). The use of metaphors also emphasizes differentiation as the key property defining stem cells. Five types of images act as the vehicle for defining stem cells: building or repair, ancestry, youth, mastery, and blank slate.

Building metaphors imply that stem cell differentiation produces all the components needed to build a body. An NBC news report in 2000 features Dr. Ron McKay, a stem cell research at the NIH, who remarks, "Stem cells construct tissues. They build other cells" ("Christopher Reeve Asks," 2000). The most common construction image is that stem cells are "building blocks." An ABC news report on the eve of President Bush's decision on funding ES cell research claims, "People like to call stem cells the building blocks of the body, and they are" ("President Bush Will Announce," 2001). A CBS report explicitly ties the image of "building blocks" to an appeal to medical applications: "These amazing stem cells are building blocks that scientists hope can cure major illnesses" ("Federal Guidelines," 2000). Images of stem cells as the producers of "spare parts"—replacements for cells and tissues that have worn out—further emphasize medical applications (see, for example, "Here's What Debate," 2001).

Ancestry metaphors emphasize that ES cells are the first cells in the body and adult stem cells are the earliest cells to appear in a tissue or organ. *The Washington Post* describes ES cells as "the most primordial of embryonic cells, each of which has the potential to grow into any kind of tissue in the body" (Weiss, 1998). A *Boston Globe* article describes a type of adult stem cell, neural stem cells, as "'progenitor' cells with offspring that can be any kind of brain cell" (Saltus, 1999). The metaphor of youth also emphasizes the temporal priority of ES cells. Wolf Blitzer tells viewers, "Stem cells are immature cells that can be made to mature into any type of body tissue" ("Wolf Blitzer Reports," 2001). In both cases, differentiation appears in the fact that these cells either have descendants or grow into mature cells constituting the body. Mastery metaphors emphasize the power of differentiation. ES cells are "these powerful cells that can become any cell or tissue type for you" ("New Technology," 2000). Tom Brokaw introduces a story on ES cell research by observing, "Stem cells are the master growth cells found in human embryos" ("Christopher Reeve Asks," 2000). Some variation of "master cell" is common (Marchione, 1999; "President Bush to Announce," 2001; Schmickle, 1999a, 2000b). These cells exhibit their mastery in the creation of the human body, in the same way that a master craftsman exhibits knowledge of his or her craft in the artifact produced. Finally, metaphors using the blank slate emphasize the ability of scientists to transform these cells into the tissues needed to cure disease. CNN's Elizabeth Cohen describes ES cells as "blank cells that can be turned into basically any type of tissue" ("President Bush Makes Decision," 2001). *The Atlanta Journal-Constitution* says, "Embryonic stem cells are basic, blank cells that can change into any one of the more than 200 specific tissue and organ types that make up the human body" (Brister, 2001), and CBS's Jane Clayson notes, "Stem cells are like blank slates which can be transformed into any kind of human tissue ("Whether Stem Cell Research" 2001).

Whether appearing as an explicit, denotative definition or through the connotations of metaphor, the stem cell's capacity for differentiation is emphasized more than self-renewal in popular discourse. This marks a shift in emphasis from scientific discourse in which the qualities of self-renewal and differentiation appeared side by side as the defining characteristics of stem cells. This shift in emphasis resulted from a change in the *kairos* of the discourse, the move to a future of new medical applications. Medical application requires stem cells to be able to become the many types of cells and tissues they will replace. While "self-renewal" might be useful, it is not as necessary as it is for research applications or pharmaceutical applications, both of which would require a constant supply of similar cells to use in experiments and testing.

Kairos not only requires working within the constraints of a situation and defining the present moment as an opportune moment for action; it also requires the creation of a future. In order to maximize the appeal to future medical applications, rhetors must present an ideal situation in which stem cell research will result in the greatest advantage—the greatest number of cures—in the quickest period of time. Rhetors must also describe the trajectory from the present to the future by providing quantitative and qualitative descriptions of that trajectory.

Creating the Future: Amplifying the Scope and Quality of Research

Rhetors make broad claims for medical applications—the future that stem cell research will bring—yet also try to avoid clarifying those claims when questioned about them. This occurs because of the tension between the act of claiming as large a relative advantage as possible and the probable (and, therefore, uncertain) nature of any possible future. Rhetors cannot guarantee that the research on which they ask Congress to spend millions of dollars will lead to the applications they claim, and the larger the claim of application, the greater the disappointment and anger will be if those applications do not appear. Yet, maximizing the future advantage of ES cell research is an important part of political discourse on stem cell research: Unlike scientific discourse which primarily asks people to believe in the research results being suggested, popular discourse focuses on federal financing for this research and demands a greater commitment from its audiences. Maximizing the advantage that will accrue from this research defines stem cells, especially ES cells, as a path to medical application too valuable to be ignored. Rhetors do two things to maximize the appearance of future advantage. First, they provide a list of diseases, many of which cannot be cured today, and argue that ES cell research will cure them. Second, they use superlative language to describe the powers of ES cells.

The appeal of medical applications gains part of its power because of the breadth of diseases that ES cell research might help cure. As Christopher Reeve once noted, "These cells have the potential to cure diseases and conditions ranging from Parkinson's and multiple sclerosis to diabetes and heart disease, Alzheimer's, Lou Gehrig's disease, even spinal-cord injuries like my own" (*Stem Cell Research, part 3,* 2000, p. 38). Many rhetors in politics and in news media provide similar lists of diseases. The diseases mentioned cover a wide spectrum of conditions: from Down's syndrome to Parkinson's and Alzheimer's disease to Huntington's disease. Some rhetors discuss only one disease: In political testimony, when only one disease is mentioned, it is always Parkinson's disease or type I diabetes, and when the news media focus on a single disease or condition, it is usually, but not always, a discussion of spinal cord injuries accompanied by an interview with Christopher Reeve (see, for example, "President Bush Makes Decision," 2001). On average, political discourses list about four diseases. Television discourse mentions just under two diseases on average, and newspapers mention just over three. The two most commonly mentioned diseases in all discourse examined are Parkinson's disease and type I diabetes. Alzheimer's disease, spinal cord injury, and heart disease make up a second tier of commonly mentioned diseases in the discourse examined. (For a complete list of diseases and the frequency of their appearance, see table 1).

The most commonly mentioned diseases are degenerative diseases that destroy cells and would require some type of replacement cell or tissue. Many of these diseases—especially Alzheimer's disease, Parkinson's disease, spinal cord injuries, and type I diabetes—have no cures at this time. References to these diseases help define ES cells as *the* path that would lead to curing them. By enumerating a list of these diseases, proponents try to maximize the advantage of pursuing ES cell research, and they define ES cells as a medical panacea. The more diseases mentioned, the greater the advantages that can come from supporting ES cell research, and the greater the difficulty in arguing *against* ES cell research.

The depiction of a future in which stem cell research leads to new medical applications is also emphasized through superlative language. Some, like Harold Varmus, describe ES cells as the key to a scientific and medical revolution: "It is not too unrealistic to say that this research has the potential to revolutionize the practice of medicine and improve the quality and length of life" (*Stem Cell Research,* 1999, p. 10). The language of revolution also appears in the testimony of Dr. Lawrence Goldstein: "The specific issue today concerns human stem cells, which have extraordinary potential to revolutionize the treatment and cure of devastating human diseases. . . . the list of possible therapeutic uses is almost endless" (*Stem Cell Research*, 1999, p. 97). Not only do stem cells constitute a medical revolution, proponents begin to represent them as a cure for everything. This superlative language for describing the future of stem cell application also appears in the news media. A CNN story on the initial scientific discovery of human ES cells claims they can "repair virtually any damaged human tissue" ("Presidential Ethics Panel," 1998). *The St. Louis Post-Dispatch* notes, "Their versatility has led some to tout the cells as the best hope to develop cures for almost any physical damage or disease that afflicts humans" (Hesman, 2001b).

Politicians and news reporters are somewhat incredulous when presented with such an optimistic view of stem cell research. After hearing Dr. Varmus's testimony about the almost limitless potential of stem cells, Sen. Arlen Specter asks him a series of questions to clarify the scope of medical application:

> SPECTER: Are there any limitations as to the range of this kind of a technique on curing diseases? Would it apply to everything?
>
> VARMUS: Well, Senator, it's a little difficult to answer the question because it is very difficult to know what science would be possible of producing. And as you've heard from the . . .
>
> SPECTER: But the basic point is you find a way of replicating cells which are diseased. So would there be any apparent limitation on the scope of these technologies to cure any kind of a disease?
>
> VARMUS: There would be certain kinds of diseases. For example, infections would not immediately be amenable to therapies with these cells. (*Stem Cell Research*, 1999, p. 26)

Specter's question reflects the testimony provided in the hearing that emphasizes the scope of stem cell application—namely, that stem cells could cure everything.[4] Varmus first tries to avoid the question. Yet, at Specter's insistence, Varmus indicates that the scope of application is quite wide and that only infectious diseases might be excluded. Although proponents define ES cells as a future medical panacea, they resist clarifying the exact scope of application. Journalists frame these concerns by highlighting that, at present, cures have been discovered only in mice. CNN's Elizabeth Cohen warns, "Now it's important to remember that this research has only showed results in rodents so far. It's not known if it will work in people" ("President Bush Makes Decision," 2001), and *The Boston Globe* offers a similar warning: "In mice, scientists have used stem cells to cure paralysis, diabetes and brain disease. This has generated enormous hope among researchers. But mouse cures do not mean human cures" (Mishra, 2001c).

Table 1. Diseases mentioned in popular discourse organized by type/media and frequency of appearance

Disease	Political Discourse	Television News	High-Impact Newspapers[a]	Low-Impact Newspapers[b]	TOTAL
Parkinson's disease	50	33	33	56	172
Type I diabetes	56	20	31	40	147
Alzheimer's disease	35	31	21	30	117
Spinal cord injury	24	19	10	32	85
Heart disease	27	8	8	28	71
Cancer	18	2	16	18	54
Stroke	10	2	2	15	29
ALS/Lou Gehrig's disease	13	3	1	7	24
Multiple sclerosis	4	3	2	7	16
"Replacement parts" (incl. all refs to organ/tissue transplant)	—	2	6	7	15
Leukemia	3	2	1	8	14
Arthritis	4	1	0	7	12
Liver disease (includes cirrhosis and hepatitis)	1	1	1	9	12
Burns	1	1	1	7	10

Paralysis	2	1	0	4	7
Sickle–cell anemia	2	1	0	3	6
Huntington's disease	0	0	2	3	5
Other diseases (incl. all diseases with less than 5 total mentions each)	8	8	2	24	42
General medical application (no disease or function mentioned)	13 (+5 neg. ref)	21	6	7	47

[a]High-impact newspapers, specifically *The New York Times* and *USA Today*, represent the most prominent and most popular newspapers in the United States during the period studied.

[b]Low-impact newspapers are newspapers from across the United States that are aimed at local or regional audiences.

In order to tie the definition of ES cells to American desires for a better (medical) future, proponents make expansive claims about the advantages people will gain from ES cell research, but the realization of those advantages is probable and not absolutely certain. This means that rhetors begin to offer caveats about the state of research, while trying to avoid attenuating the advantage they have associated with support of ES cell research.

Establishing a Trajectory to the Future: Creating Timelines for Medical Application

The request for federal funding for ES cell research necessitates making promises on when the government and the American people can get a return on their investment: American pragmatism requires some assurance as to *when* benefits from the research will appear. The quicker the return, the greater the support provided. Rhetors therefore must emphasize the expediency of this research. Rhetors declare that the trajectory from the present state of research on ES cells to the realization of cures is relatively short, typically five to ten years. Proponents define ES cells as the quickest means to producing cures for a number of diseases. This definition depends on an ideal presentation of scientific progress: It assumes a best-case scenario of experimentation, but that best-case scenario becomes qualified as the debate about stem cell research progresses. Two timelines—five to ten years and ten to twenty years—are established in the first hearing on stem cell research in 1998. Later political testimony emphasizes the shorter timeline, while news reports emphasize the longer timeline. Both political and news discourse identify situational factors that can impede the advancement of ES cell research and present those factors as caveats to the timeline given. These caveats embody the places where proponents manage the limits of their current situation and its potential to attenuate the *kairos* they craft around ES cell research. Political caveats characterize situational factors impeding research as external to science and controlled by politicians, while news caveats describe scientific ignorance of ES cells as the factor most likely to impede progress.

Political timelines. The first round of testimony on ES cell research establishes the timelines used to discuss medical applications in public discourse. Scientists at that hearing claim that ES cell research will lead to cures "soon," but they do not provide an explicit time. One of the boldest claims comes from Dr. Thomas Okarma: "In conclusion, the therapeutic applications of this technology are real and near term" (*Stem Cell Research,* 1999, p. 52). Okarma establishes that ES cell research is an expedient means of curing many diseases. Dr. James Thomson also provides a general timeframe, but his timeframe places medical applications somewhat farther in the future. Near the beginning of his testimony, he notes, "Although the long-term potential for human therapies resulting from human ES cell line research is enormous, these therapies will take years to develop. Significant advances in developmental biology and transplantation medicine are required, but I believe that therapies resulting from human ES cell research will become available within my lifetime. How soon such therapies will be developed will depend on whether there is public support of research in this area" (*Stem Cell Research,* 1999, p. 16). In contrast to Okarma, Thomson provides a nuanced view of the challenges and timeframe within which medical therapies based on stem cells will develop. The possibility of medical applications of ES cell research is long-term and requires significant scientific and medical advances. Such advances require public support and funding, but Thomson believes they will be developed in his lifetime.

In both examples, no exact number of years is provided. After the initial testimony, Senators Specter and Harkin begin to question the scientists and NIH director Harold Varmus about these timelines for producing cures. Specter, especially, asks for a specific, narrow timeline for one particular disease, Parkinson's disease. The focus on one disease forces scientists to clarify their answers instead of talking about cures for ambiguous numbers of diseases in an ambiguous future. Scientists provide a range of years within which cures might appear, but they also expand on the caveat Thomson provided in his initial timeline: Public support is necessary to realize the future the scientists portray.

Specter asks his question of all the scientists at the hearing. The interchange between Senator Specter and Dr. John Gearhart is representative of these exchanges and the issues raised:

SPECTER: Dr. Gearhart, what kind of a time line do you see on the kind of research you have done to provide practical answers to problems like Parkinson's or Alzheimer's or cancer?

GEARHART: Actually, I think Parkinson's will be one of the first targets and one that we will see in a short period.

SPECTER: How long is a short period?

GEARHART: Well, now let me back off.

SPECTER: No, no. Go on.

GEARHART: I will. I actually think within several years to be honest with you, because these neurons that I have demonstrated here, we don't know, to be honest, since this is new data, we do not know what neurons they represent, what type, whether they are cholinergic, dopaminergic, etc. (*Stem Cell Research,* 1999, p. 32)

Gearhart first indicates that cures for Parkinson's disease will appear shortly. When Specter asks for clarification, Gearhart initially resists providing an answer, but after further prodding, he says a cure for Parkinson's disease will appear in several years. He then provides a new caveat that the neurons produced by ES cells require further study: The current state of ES cell research with neurons does not provide a sufficient foundation for a short timeline to cures. Like Gearhart, all the speakers during this initial hearing hesitate before providing a more exact answer. While they have portrayed a near-term future of wondrous medical advancements that is the result of ES cell research, the trajectory toward any future is always indeterminate and uncertain. The uncertainty about what is required, or possible, to achieve an imagined future makes offering a confident answer about when it will arrive problematic.

Already in these initial exchanges, scientists have begun to qualify the trajectory—the timeline—along which medical applications can be expected. They deflect attention away from lacunae in scientific knowledge about ES cells and claim that public funding of the research will determine when cures appear. The scientists' answers to Senator Harkin's line of questioning continue this trend:

> HARKIN: Let me focus a little bit—now, you talked about this time line that the chairman just laid down in terms of Parkinson's. What I basically heard was that anywhere from three to five to 12 years, somewhere in there we might be finding something. Is that assuming the federal ban continues and this research is not allowed to go forward . . . If this federal ban is deemed to cover research on stem cells, does your time line hold?
>
> MICHAEL WEST: This time line I gave, seven to 12 years for Parkinson's, assumed that the NIH would be allowed to fund research in differentiating these cells into cells for Parkinson's.
>
> HARKIN: So your answers were based on . . .
>
> WEST: Yes.
>
> HARKIN [continuing]: I should not say lifting the ban, because, see, I don't think the ban applies.
>
> WEST: Right.
>
> HARKIN: So I have got to be careful about what I say. So your time line is based upon an interpretation or reading of this that the ban does not apply to stem cell research.
>
> WEST: Right.
>
> HARKIN: Is that true of all of you?
>
> VARMUS: That is correct.
>
> THOMSON: That is correct, but also the number of diseases likely to be

treated will increase exponentially if there is public funding. (*Stem Cell Research,* 1999, p.33)

If a future where stem cells lead to cures for Parkinson's disease is to be realized, scientists claim that the NIH must fund this research. A condition has been set on realizing the potential of stem cells to produce medical therapies quickly. If the cures are not achieved, proponents of ES cell research can blame the federal government or the public for the failure to attain cures.

This testimony sets the pattern for subsequent political discussion of time-lines for stem cell research. Scientists try to provide a general claim that stem cell research will produce cures in a relatively short period of time. Politicians push for specific answers, and scientists dodge the question or qualify their previous answers. Scientists characterize the impediments to realizing cures as external to scientific research and under the control of Congress and the federal government. The timeline and related caveats reflect the situational constraint of funding and deflect attention from the fact that the research is still in its infancy while helping to manage an uncertain and indeterminate future. The possibility that the research will fail to lead to cures is transformed into an external impediment to research, implying that scientists will succeed if given sufficient funding.

From late 1998 until the end of 2001, proponents of ES cell research confidently provide their timelines and argue that sufficient federal funding will make a hoped-for future of medical applications possible. Scientists base these time-lines on an idealistic vision of scientific progress. Occasionally, these assumptions are brought to light. For example, then–NIH director Harold Varmus notes, "And there are experimental models, especially in mice, that indicate that certain other tissues, like the heart, may be repaired. . . . Given those precedents, it seems to me that within the course of the next decade or two, with an appropriate cadre of investigators, that many, many diseases would be at least treated, if not entirely cured, by the kind of cell therapies we are talking about" (*Stem Cell Research,* 1999, p. 28). Varmus provides a ten- to twenty-year timeline during which "many, many diseases" will be cured, but that timeline assumes that certain precedents from mouse research hold and that "appropriate" scientists conduct the work. These assumptions become even more explicit in the September 2000 question-and-answer exchange between Senator Specter and Dr. Darwin Prockop:

SPECTER: What do you anticipate in two to three years with respect to stem cells and Parkinson's?
PROCKOP: Well, I can give you the best case scenario. If our experi-

ments now being conducted in animals come out right in terms of efficacy, in toxicity, we think we may be able to begin the very first clinical trials in patients with Parkinsonism in two or three years. That's a best case scenario.

SPECTER: Why not sooner, Dr. Prockop?

PROCKOP: Senator Specter, we have to be safe about this. We have to be sure we are not going to do more damage than we are going to help the patients.

. . . .

SPECTER: Well, you are going to have to qualify with the Food and Drug Administration, understandably so, important precautions, but my question goes to do you have a projection as to how long it will take to cure Parkinson's?

PROCKOP: Senator Specter, I am an optimist, all right? One has to be an optimist to do research. I think it's somewhere in the order of four or five years. I'm saying it is two or three years for the first few patients, carefully controlled studies and a very carefully controlled environment. I am hoping it goes fast after that. (*Stem Cell Research, part 3,* 2000, pp. 90–91).

Specter pushes Prockop to provide a prediction on where research on a stem cell–based cure for Parkinson's disease will be in three years, and he treats FDA requirements as an obvious part of medical research that does not impact his question. In his answer, Prockop notes that he is an "optimist" before rearticulating the five-year timeline that first appeared in 1998. He grounds his optimism and the timeline in an ideal vision of science, where scientific progress, the journey from the earliest experiments to full-blown medical applications, occurs rapidly.

After President Bush allows funding for some ES cell research, scientists do not paint so rosy a picture of science. The fundamental uncertainty underlying any research program is no longer deflected, partly because, with funding available for research, the public might demand the timeline be honored. In December 2001, Dr. West balks at answering a question about when medical applications will appear: "You're asking a question that scientists always hesitate to answer, you know, it's so hard to predict the future of science and how fast things will develop because they aren't all in our control" (*Cloning 2001,* 2001, pp. 37–38). West does not provide a timeframe based on the best-case scenario of science. Instead, prediction becomes difficult, if not impossible, because so much is outside the individual scientist's control. Thomas Murray, of the Hastings Center, expresses a more explicit concern about the progress of stem cell research: "One observation that I would like to make is that it is very difficult to predict the course of the science. It is impossible to predict with any confidence exactly where the science will go, even if it will ever lead to useful therapies. But of course, we will never know unless we try" (*Dangers of Cloning,* 2002, p. 39). With Murray's comments, the possibility of medical applications itself becomes uncertain. The uncertainty of the future becomes the basis for refusing to speculate about when ES cell research will produce results. Yet, despite this uncertainty about science's progress, Murray claims that research must still continue. For the majority of this debate, scientists emphasize the shorter timeline because the *kairos* of political discussion requires crafting the present moment as the "right time" for financial support. This lack of financial support becomes the "untimely" action that delays the future proponents depict. When financial support, however limited, becomes available after August 2001, scientists then argue that the impossibility of predicting the future renders any prediction problematic.

News timelines. Uncertainty about the state of science and its ability to achieve progress is the main qualification to the timelines provided in journalistic discourse. Only a few news reports include a short timeline. The shortest timeline presented—two years for human clinical trials—focuses on a well-studied set of neural stem cells, not ES cells (Saltus, 2000). Only one article rearticulates the caveats about external impediments to realizing medical applications: "Some treatments could be ready within five years, but only with government support, said Dr. James Thomson" (Associated Press, 1998). The only other news article to mention five years as a realistic timeframe for medical applications includes a number of caveats:

> In reality, we know surprisingly little about stem cells. Fundamental questions remain: What is the mechanism by which they specialize? How can we control what they become? How can we deliver them to patients with precision?
>
> Even if stem cell research takes off in the coming years, researchers estimate it will be at least five years before the first clinical tests begin. And many of these will fail. (Mishra, 2001c)

Clinical tests might appear in five years, but present scientific questions and the specter of future experimental failure haunt this prediction. The nature of scientific research—the failure of many clinical trials—comes to the fore in journalistic discourse on ES cells.

Typically, journalists present timelines of ten years or more, which is in line with the specific timeline provided by Dr. Harold Varmus in his testimony to

Congress, rather than the shorter timelines provided by other scientists. A CBS reporter claims, "we have a long way to go" before medical applications appear ("Federal Guidelines," 2000), and *The Atlanta Journal-Constitution* says that "using stem cells to treat patients is far down the road" (Brister, 2001). ABC's medical editor Timothy Johnson claims, "The ultimate goal of growing entire organs that can be transplanted, I guess, must be decades away" ("Enormous Scientific Breakthrough," 1998). Minneapolis's *Star Tribune* declares, "Patients aren't likely to benefit from much of the research for at least a decade" (Schmickle, 1999b).

While political discourse by proponents of ES cell research claims that science will develop medical applications quickly unless hindered by the government and lack of financial support, journalistic discussion of when medical applications appear describes the state of ES cell research as the primary hindrance. "Human tests of stem cell therapies are probably years away, largely because scientists know so little about the cells," claims a *Washington Post* article (Gillis & Connolly, 2001). *The Star Tribune* notes, "The lessons from the early research are that the applications will come more slowly than expected" (Schmickle, 2000b). CNN closes a report on stem cell research with the following: "If the experiments move forward without complications, researchers estimate that it would take 10 to 15 years to begin using the cells to treat disease. The question is what medical and ethical complications might arise" ("Presidential Ethics Panel," 1998).

The journalistic discussion of when cures will appear reflects the differences between a scientistic idiom and scientific rhetoric. A scientistic idiom is not dependent on any specific scientific claim, and it can transform scientific claims into issues where debate and uncertainty exist. Journalistic discussion of a timeframe uses the longer of the two timeframes first presented to Congress in 1998, rather than the shorter timeline used by scientists and other proponents in later political discourse. Journalists also describe the state of ES cell research—the lack of knowledge about stem cells, the lessons of early research, and uncertainty about the results of future experiments—as a reason why medical applications will develop slowly. Because the journalists are not directly advocating for this research and are not beholden to the scientists who speak to Congress, the state of scientific research becomes a topic for discussion.

The Power and Pitfalls of "Promise"

In addition to describing a future in which many diseases are cured and outlining the trajectory, or timeframe, that will lead to this future, scientific and popular rhetors both turn to the language of "promise" to lend certainty to the uncertain prospect of stem cell research and its future applications. Yet, using the language of "promise" has risks. Emphasizing the opportunity—the "promise"—in the moment always already raises the possibility of failure. The uncertainty of the future means that despite attempts at containing uncertainty and the perception of failure, opponents can still raise these issues. This becomes clearest in the discussion of stem cell research's "promise." While initially used in a positive fashion, "promise" contains an ambivalent thread. Some proponents use that ambivalence to warn against promising too much, too soon, and opponents use it to argue that medical applications of ES cell research are illusory or ephemeral, especially when compared to current uses of alternative stem cell sources.

Positive uses of promise language almost always refer to ES cell research and its possible medical applications. Bioethicist Arthur Caplan argues that stem cell research "holds the promise of allowing the development of techniques for manipulating, growing and cloning these cells to permit the creation of designer cells and tissues" (*Stem Cell Research,* 1999, p. 37). The prepared testimony of Drs. Allen Spiegel and Gerald Fischbach argues, "Research using human pluripotent stem cells holds enormous promise for advances in the prevention, treatment and diagnosis of a vast array of diseases" (*Stem Cell Research, part 3,* 2000, p. 5). Similar language appears in journalistic discourse. A *USA Today* article says stem cell research "is regarded as one of the most promising fields of research" (Friend, 2001f), and *The New York Times* notes that ES cells "hold promise for treating Type I diabetes" (Wade, 2001c). Stem cell research presents the opportunity, the "promise," for curing diseases, especially diseases for which no cures exist. Some news reports weave the language of promise into a story of individuals who could benefit from the potential medical applications in order to buttress the appeal to application. A CBS news report begins with an image of muscular sclerosis sufferer Steve Moritz: "Everyday Steve Moritz thinks about the promise of stem cell research. He has muscular sclerosis, making it a struggle to play with his children and a fight to climb stairs. He can't understand why anyone would oppose using stem cells to cure this degenerative disease" ("Scientists and Anti-Abortion Activists," 2001). A CNN report shows a young diabetic girl talking to legislators on the steps of the Capitol: "12-year-old Mollie and Jackie Singer skipped a vacation to come to Washington. Mollie has juvenile diabetes. . . . She says research on stem cells offers promise for a cure" ("Stem Cell Research," 2001). In both cases, the potential to cure diseases is brought down from an abstract level of "diseases" to specific diseases and individual sufferers. Appeals for ES cell research are also harder to resist when they are tied to specific individuals, since opposing these people's desire for a cure can be interpreted as a willingness to ignore the suffering of others.

Despite the use of "promise" to emphasize the positive aspects of ES cell research, "promise" describes something that is only potential waiting to be realized. Some advocates use this ambiguity in the word to recognize and manage the uncertainty surrounding ES cell research. This is the basis for the following counterintuitive statement by Dr. David Korn: "The promise is real because of the enormous capability of these cells, and we've never had that potential in medicine or biology before" ("Controversy Brewing," 2001). Promise, in this case, is "real" yet it is still a potential waiting to be realized. Korn tries to strengthen the appeal to potential by presenting it as real or actual. Usually supporters who discuss the uncertain nature of promise do so as a warning against overselling the possibility of future medical applications. Dr. James Childress tells the Senate Committee on Health, Education, Labor and Pensions, "We must carefully scrutinize claims of scientific promise, being wary of unfounded optimism, but we must not neglect research that offers a significant prospect of major medical breakthroughs that may alleviate human suffering and reduce the number of premature deaths" (*Stem Cell Research,* 2001, p. 74). Childress presents a two-sided argument, warning against unfounded optimism yet saying that the promise, or potential, of stem cell research to cure disease is quite great. Sen. Bill Frist (R-TN) offers a similar warning to Congress at the same hearing: "Yet I think we need to be very, very careful at this juncture, early in our discussions—and yes indeed, it is early in the evolution of this relatively new science—not to oversell the promise of this research to the American people" (*Stem Cell Research,* 2001, p. 7). Frist recognized the situational constraint that human ES cell research began only a few years before he spoke. His recognition of that fact is offered as a warning to fellow legislators against overselling the promise of ES cell research.

Similar warnings appear in the media. The first type of warning highlights the fact that research has shown cures only in mice. *The Houston Chronicle* notes, "Still, for all the talk, the only real proof of stem cells' effectiveness so far involves rats and mice" (Ackerman, 2001). CNN's Elizabeth Cohen warns viewers, "Now it's important to remember that this research has only showed results in rodents so far. It's not known if it will work in people" ("President Bush Makes Decision," 2001). The most extensive warning of this type appears in an exchange between ABC's Charles Gibson and medical correspondent Dr. Timothy Johnson:

> GIBSON: A lot of this, Tim, is still theoretical, and I'm interested whether you think the scientists can do with stem cells what a lot of them predict they can do. I mean, is it practical reality, or is it science fiction?
> JOHNSON: Oh, it's much closer, I think, to reality than science fiction. This potential—not certain promise, but potential—is based on very good laboratory research with animals, and it has a lot of good hints

that it will work in humans. I think it holds enormous potential to be one of the great discoveries of medicine of all time. ("Dr. Tim Johnson Explains," 2001)

Gibson highlights that medical applications are theoretical and that the promises are so great they border on science fiction. Johnson clarifies the issue in his assertion that the promise is "real," but he complicates his assessment of stem cell research by dissociating promises into those that provide certitude and those that denote potential. This rhetorical balancing act occurs because the medical applications have been researched only in animals and not humans. Warnings of this type try to balance creating hope for cures that will drive public support and ultimately public funding with the situational constraints of limited experimental evidence and research that has not gone beyond animal studies.

A second set of warnings emphasizes that rhetors in the stem cell debate have overemphasized the possibility of medical applications: While the promise is there, "too much" has been promised. The argument here recognizes the state of ES cell science as a constraint on rhetoric that has been ignored by previous rhetors. A *Washington Post* article describes the concerns of some scientists about recent reports on adult stem cell research: "Some criticized the publicity surrounding the newest work as representative of a worrisome trend of overselling the medical and financial promise of a research field still in its infancy" (Weiss, 2000b). Another article reports that scientists "worry that stem-cell therapy has been so overhyped it cannot help but disappoint" (Ackerman, 2001). *USA Today* attributes the "hyperbole" around stem cell research to the political debate and the actions of both proponents and opponents: "Proponents have exaggerated the potential benefits, while detractors have exaggerated the benefits of using adult stem cells instead" (Friend, 2001a). Finally, *The New York Times* reports that scientists explain their actions against the backdrop of the political debate: "But with calls by some politicians to ban the work, and to bar any use of tax money to pay for it, scientists say they feel obliged to stress how important the research is. And, some say, they now fear they may have promised too much" (Kolata, 2001). These warnings highlight a complex situation. Science requires public funding, but science dealing with controversial topics, like embryos and fetuses, must overcome serious obstacles. Promising applications does that, but it requires extrapolating from animal studies and preliminary research with human cells. These warnings attempt to rein in the promises and the enthusiasm they generate. The majority of the articles describe this as a general feature of "publicity" or the give-and-take of political debate, but the *New York Times* article identifies *scientists* as the guilty party in overselling the potential of stem cell research. Yet, while it does so, it also highlights justification for making such promises, namely that opposition by politicians has necessitated these promises. The promises that have been made have become "untimely" by promising too much, too soon, thus guaranteeing that stem cell research will disappoint the public in the future. Ironically, these untimely promises have become the timely situation for warnings about the public rhetoric of ES cell research and for attempts to manage and reduce expectations for it.

The majority of references to the "promise" of stem cell research emphasize the positive elements: Promise implies that individuals will work hard to make this promise a reality in the future. Yet, promises are often broken. Sometimes a promise is broken because the trajectory from current promise to future application does not exist: In this case, studies in mice might mislead us to believe the promise that human medical applications exist when they in fact do not. The breaking of a promise might also lead to an individual to be blamed: Present-day scientists are often indicted in the newspaper coverage for promising too much.

Opposition Use of "Promise" and *Kairos*

Finally, the uncertainty of "promise" and "potential" becomes the basis for opposing ES cell research. The uncertainty of *kairos,* whether presented as a "promise" or some other rhetorical figure, opens up the possibility that as proponents try to seize the advantage of the "right time" they also create the "right time" for their opposition to attack. Furthermore, the uncertainty that makes the timing of the original support for ES cell research possible also becomes a resource to be used in arguing against that research and trying to undermine attempts at linking ES cell research to the American desire for a better future and to help the medically disadvantaged.

Opponents explicitly use the language of promise to oppose ES cell research only a handful of times. Dr. Christopher Hook asks, "Are we willing to set the precedent that the promise, not proof, of future medical treatments for third party patients is sufficient to endorse the destruction of living human beings now?" (*Opportunities and Advancements,* 2001, p. 175). Hook contrasts "promise" with "proof"—since ES cells have not actually produced medical applications, pursuing research on ES cells is not justifiable, especially since it requires the destruction of embryos. The testimony of 16-year-old Eric Salley, who underwent a transfusion of hematopoietic stem cells from umbilical cord blood to treat leukemia, directs the language of "promise" away from ES cells to adult stem cells: "I'm living proof that there are promising and useful alternatives to embryonic stem cell research and that embryos do not need to be killed to achieve medical breakthroughs" (*Opportunities and Advancements,* 2001, p. 97). Salley uses his treatment and its success to claim that adult stem cells show greater promise than ES cells: His presence at the hearing embodies that promise.

In addition to the language of promise, other means have been used to secure the image of the future and the trajectory leading to it, and these strategies are also critiqued. For example, Rep. Dave Weldon (R–FL) attacks the future proposed by proponents directly: "It's science fiction . . . . To hold this out
as the viable solution to all these terrible health problems is very disingenuous"
(Friend, 2001b). Direct attacks like this are extremely rare: Nothing similar appeared in the political or news discourse that was examined. Other direct attacks focus on the trajectory from present potential to future application that
proponents envision. Dr. Anton-Lewis Usala argues, "While many respected scientists are understandably enthused about the possibilities, human embryonic
stem cells may not provide a viable path [to therapies]" (*Stem Cell Research, part
3,* 2000, p. 99). Usala uses a spatial metaphor to trouble the trajectory from present promise to future application: ES cells might appear like a "path" leading to
a cure, but that possibility might be a dead end. Father Kevin Fitzgerald makes
a comparison between the expediency and advantage provided by ES cell research and other scientific avenues: "It may well be the case that for many patients the treatments for their illnesses may come more quickly from research
avenues other than human embryonic stem cell research, and that these alternative treatments may even be better than any treatment derived from human
embryonic stem cell research" (*Stem Cell Research,* 2001, p. 78). Fitzgerald tries
to attack the *kairos* of ES cell research, claiming that other research avenues will
lead to a better future (in other words, more applications) and will do so more
quickly than ES cell research, but his claim leaves murky the image of the present opportunity that will lead to this future. Finally, Sen. Judd Gregg (R–NH)
describes the present state of adult stem cell research as more advantageous than
the future promised by ES cell research: "These therapies, unlike the unproven
and untested potential application of embryonic stem cell therapies, which are
at minimum 5 and potentially 10 years away from clinical application, are actually being used today, and are being used very successfully, and we should not
forget that" (*Stem Cell Research,* 2001, pp. 4–5). According to Gregg, ES cells
compare unfavorably to adult stem cells. Using the same timeline established by
James Thomson in 1998, Gregg claims that medical applications from ES cells
will be at least five years away, while therapies based on adult stem cells already
exist. Gregg's description also contrasts the potential and the actual: ES cell research is only potential waiting to be proven, while adult stem cells offer actual
cures right now.

Kairos and Promise in Stem Cells and Science

Conjectures, like the potential applications of ES cells, shape the range of real
definitions. A focus on application makes research in the present moment the

ideal time and space for realizing a future of new scientific breakthroughs and medical cures facilitated by ES cell research if only scientists and politicians foster it. *Kairos,* with its focus on the "right time" for action, is the rhetorical principle that highlights this quality in definitions of ES cells. These definitions make the isolation of ES cells an opportunity to realize a number of applications for scientists and various publics, but scientific and popular rhetors must also tailor their responses to account for the fact that the research is just beginning and that ongoing research continues to shape our understanding of ES cells.

Kairos and application act as a key definitional strategy, but the range of applications shifts when discourse about ES cells moves from the technical sphere to the public sphere. The narrowed range of applications reflects the move from scientific discourse to the public's scientistic idiom. While the scientistic idiom draws broadly from scientific styles of argument and discourse, it operates independently of any specific scientific argument or claim. Thus, the scientific arguments for research and pharmaceutical applications disappear in broad, scientistic appeals to a general public. This also alters the way in which the *kairotic* moment is presented. Scientific presentation of the research, pharmaceutical, and medical applications aims to create *belief* in scientific audiences that the isolation of ES cells creates the opportunity to further numerous scientific projects. Popular presentation in Congressional testimony and journalistic discourse aims to create financial support for this research. Because of this, popular discourse about stem cell research must go to greater lengths to convince audiences, such as enumerating the advantages and expediency of the research as well as trying to minimize the uncertainty about the opportune moment and future application through the language of promise. Furthermore, the *type* of future presented, specifically which applications are discussed, determines what qualities found in the present moment are defined as key to achieving the future opportunity. For scientific discourse with its equal emphasis on all three applications, "self-renewal" and "differentiation" are key, while political discourse's emphasis on medical applications over the others means that "differentiation" becomes emphasized in numerous ways.

The *kairos* of stem cell research is powerful, regardless of its deployment as advantage, expediency, or promise. The creation of what Carolyn Miller has called "opportunities for opportunity" works because the image of a better future is a powerful enticement (1994, p. 93). Yet these claims must be balanced against the limitations of scientific knowledge and the limits on federal funding. Some rhetors found the promise of stem cells was potentially overplayed. This should highlight that engendering hope for a better future is a powerful but double-edged sword. In describing the pressure on President Bush to support stem cell research, one commentator noted, "Whether stem cell research is really going to address these problems or not, it represents hope. And when you mess with people's hope, you're playing with fire" ("President Bush Says," 2001). Hope is a powerful emotion helping to drive support for stem cell research. The image of terrible diseases being cured because of stem cell research creates a powerful incentive to support this research.

Even if the hope should be misplaced in this case, the use of *kairos* in science and technology is grounded in it, which means that these types of appeals will always be a major strategy for tying real definitions to American ideology long after the stem cell debate ends. The hope for a better future is a powerful lure and a common refrain in American history. Although the *kairotic,* hoped-for future will always be part of a scientist idiom, it has the potential to harm specific individuals and research programs that abuse it. If stem cell research is really "oversold," then those making the sale risk being attacked and repudiated by the very public that first believed them. The use of *kairos* involves risk for the rhetor. The example of gene therapy, which experienced early, high-publicity failures leading to lost funding and credibility, highlights the risks involved when technology advocates appeal to hope.

While proponents take a risk in appealing to hope, opponents take risks in attacking it. To attack the appeal to future medical applications is to attack the hopes of the people opponents wish to persuade. This might also explain why opponents rarely offer a direct refutation of the claims for medical applications. When the language of hope can be deployed in a debate, the advantage goes to the side using it, and that side usually consists of proponents of new technology. No simple, single line of argument exists for the opposition. Instead, opponents must supplement any attack on the potential of ES cell research, or a similar scientific breakthrough, with additional lines of argument in order to make their case.

3
Abortion and the Embryo

Right-to-Life Arguments as a Source for Rhetorical Invention

Opponents of ES cell research have a difficult time challenging the language of future medical applications and its innate appeal to hope. Attacking the hope of curing Alzheimer's disease and Parkinson's disease is quixotic at best. Instead, opponents deploy other lines of argument to dissuade people from supporting ES cell research. Because ES cell research deals with the beginnings of human life, one readily available resource for opponents as well as journalists covering this debate is the cultural history of abortion in the United States. Journalists define the abortion debate as the Burkean *scene* wherein the action of the ES cell debate takes place (Burke, 1969b). Opponents use the resources of the abortion debate to define ES cells so that they appear in a negative light.

These uses of right-to-life arguments can shift public argument from a scientistic to a Manichean idiom. A Manichean idiom creates dichotomous categories and allows for no middle ground. This complicates the use of right-to-life arguments for both journalists and opponents of the research in several ways. First, prominent pro-life politicians, like Orrin Hatch and Bill Frist, support ES cell research, thus muddying the division between "good" objections (and those voicing them) and "evil" research (and those who practice it). Journalists must account for this division within the movement even as they frame the ES cell debate as an extension of debates over abortion. Pro-life opponents must address the division within their movement in order to maintain the integrity of the inventional resources they use to tackle ES cell research.

Second, this move toward a Manichean idiom can be problematic for opponents since the creation of real definitions resides in a scientistic idiom. Science and the scientistic idiom establish what counts as real for many public debates, but the pro-life movement is perceived as religiously motivated. This makes it challenging to translate pro-life objections to ES cell research into an idiom open to anyone, regardless of religious affiliation. Framing an issue as science versus religion can be very effective, as can be seen in the opposition to teaching evolution, but evolution is divorced from practical outcomes, like curing disease, in ways that ES cell research is not.[1] Insofar as medical applications are treated as a *fact,* pro-life objections, especially their association with religion, will appear as opinion or value statements that do not comport with the "reality" of stem cell research and its promise. Furthermore, even if a Manichean idiom were effective in generally framing ES cell research, the prominent defectors from the pro-life camp on this issue create the impression that ES cell research can be moral within a pro-life framework.

Finally, arguments by opponents are complicated by developments in some scientific and cultural practices. Practices involving in vitro fertilization (IVF) and determining fetal death for epidemiological studies have troubled the use of the "public fetus," which is the central rhetorical figure of right-to-life arguments. The arguments used in the abortion debate do not easily transfer from discussions of late-term fetuses with their obvious visual similarity to actual people to the earliest stages of human life, which do not appear obviously human. Opponents must explicitly extend the rights of actual humans to the 14-day-old blastocyst from which ES cells are derived.

In describing debates about this research, journalists must either deflect attention away from prominent defectors in the pro-life camp or deploy rhetorical figures that can account for them while maintaining the integrity of abortion as the scene that renders the debate intelligible. Opponents must reinvent their arguments. Specifically, they must extend the public fetus to earlier, embryonic forms of human life, while also trying to recast their objections in a scientistic idiom to define ES cells as a direct harm to developing human life.

Setting the Scene: Using Abortion to Make Sense of the Stem Cell Controversy

Journalistic coverage of the ES cell debate aims to explain what is happening in a technologically and scientifically complex area. Among the issues they seek to explain are the objections to the research. To do that, journalists emphasize the scene: They explain the action and agents in the ES cell debate against the backdrop of the abortion issue. This does not mean that journalists have chosen abortion from a set of equally likely options for explaining this issue without bias or preconception. Rather, the articulation of this issue as an *extension of the abortion debate* has implications for what becomes newsworthy and thus reported to the public. Scenes contain the acts and agents: If one knows the scene, then one understands the positions and attitudes taken (Burke, 1969a, pp. 3–9).

Yet, making abortion the scene upon which the ES cell debate plays out turns the issue into a battle between religion and science. Using abortion as the scene for this debate requires some journalists and politicians to negotiate the disparity between understanding the ES cell debate as another front in the cultural battle over abortion and the fact that some pro-life politicians support ES cell research. While abortion provides a familiar ground upon which to place the figures in the new and uncertain ES cell debate, the use of abortion as the scene that renders opposition intelligible also reduces the scope of objections to ES cell research viewed as important or legitimate. While the use of embryos is a salient issue in this debate, ethicists and scientists have identified additional ethical concerns. These other ethical issues include the commodification of human beings, overselling the potential of ES cell research, questions about who will benefit from ES cell research, and broader concerns about research priorities in biomedicine (The President's Council on Bioethics, 2004). A focus solely on abortion obfuscates these issues.

Journalistic Uses of Abortion as Scene

Journalists must try to make the ES cell debate intelligible to a public that might not have familiarity with the issue, especially when ES cells were first isolated by scientists. The news coverage studied includes 103 television news segments aired from 1998 to 2005 that were stored at the Vanderbilt Television News Archive and a sample of 200 newspaper stories from 1998 to 2002 identified through a search of the LEXIS-NEXIS news database. In that sample of news coverage, 28 out of 103 television news segments and 35 out of 200 newspaper articles place the debate within the context of abortion. Many articles and news segments use abortion in a straightforward fashion to render the situation intelligible: Opposition to ES cell research can be explained through reference to the abortion debate. This scene-setting occurs in three ways.

First, journalistic accounts most often provide a simple report that pro-life/anti-abortion groups oppose the research without supplying background information. *USA Today* claims, "The lines tend to fall along the same fronts as the abortion debate" (Friend, 2001e). In a story on contemporary advances in ES cell research, *The Seattle Times* notes, "The recent news has centered on embryonic stem cells, prompting abortion-like debates about the starting point of life" (King, 2001). Some claims go further than noting the similarity between abortion and ES cell debates by tying the debates about abortion directly to political battles over funding the research. An ABC News report from late April 2000 links the lack of funding for this research specifically to concern about abortion: "The federal government is not spending any money on this research. The federal guidelines outlining how to do it and who can do it are unfinished, the victim of political wrangling having to do with abortion" ("Controversy over Stem Cell Research," 2000). A May 2001 article in *USA Today* says, "Medical advocacy groups have formed alliances to support such research, while groups opposed to abortion and experiments on embryos have fought to stop it" (Friend, 2001h), and NBC's Brian Williams describes stem cell research as a combination of "life and death, morality and abortion, and a heavy dose of politics" ("Jones Institute Recruits," 2001). These blanket references to pro-life opposition foreground the political elements of this debate. The funding is a victim of "political wrangling," and morality is flavored with "a heavy dose of politics." This type of scene-setting defines the opposition to ES cell research as the product of religiously inflected political groups, with no connection to scientific concerns. The reasons for this maneuvering are to be inferred by viewers and readers, and such inferences are likely to make opponents' later attempts to use a scientistic idiom difficult.

The second strategy emphasizes the moral, instead of the political, nature of the opposition to ES cell research and often involves a description of pro-life principles. A CNN report in August 2000 notes, "Anti-abortion groups are opposed to the research saying it is morally wrong" ("Science/Stem Cell Research," 2000). *The St. Louis Post-Dispatch* provides a greater degree of explanation: "Abortion opponents oppose research with stem cells from embryonic tissue because they believe life begins at conception—when the sperm fertilizes the egg" (Hesman, 2001a). A similar observation appears in *The New York Times:* "Opponents of abortion have objected to federal approval of such research because the embryos, which they consider to be capable of life, are destroyed in the process" (Wade, 2000a), and Carl Hall (2001) of *The San Francisco Chronicle* notes that for pro-life individuals "the research amounts to the taking of a human life—wrong, regardless of medical value." News coverage that uses this strategy highlights the moral nature of pro-life objections. This moves the debate from the level of political wrangling to a debate about the ethical principles that should guide decisions about this research—the welfare of patients or the welfare of the unborn.

The third straightforward application amplifies the moral aspect of the debate by directly comparing ES cell research to abortion. An early newspaper report on the isolation of ES cells claims, "The latest advance hasn't convinced opponents they should put aside their ethical concerns. Anti-abortion activists are joined by many mainstream religions, which make no distinction between abortion and embryo research" ("Embryo Research Debated," 1998). *The Denver Post* in 2000 notes, "Opponents of using discarded embryos to harvest stem cells have based their arguments on their belief that life begins at the moment of conception. Researchers who harvest cells from frozen four- or five-day-old embryos, thus destroying them, are then committing an act of abortion, in this view" (Nelson, 2000). Abortion and ES cell research are considered identical from this perspective, and the comparison of ES cell research and abortion occurs even more frequently in the 2001 coverage of the debate, especially in coverage by *USA Today* and NBC ("Controversy Surrounding," 2001; "Debate over Stem Cell Research," 2001; Friend, 2001a, 2001c; Kiely, 2001a).[2]

All three of these strategies make the abortion debate the scene within which the ES cell debate occurs. This scene focuses on the moral and political nature of the opposition and involves a direct comparison of ES cells and embryos: While the ES cell research is opposed politically by abortion opponents, they do so because of their moral stand that rejects any practice that ends embryonic life or because they view ES cell research as another form of abortion. Making the political and ethical debate about abortion the scene for the ES cell debate turns the debate into a proxy for the cultural struggle over abortion.

Such scene-setting has three effects. First, by most often focusing on political wrangling and the political opposition to abortion and ES cell research, journalistic coverage transforms the ES cell debate into a story in which the issues of evidence and support for one's argument are secondary to maintaining a balance of the political positions represented in the story, regardless of their merit. Journalists addressing these issues are just as likely to be political reporters as they are to be science reporters. The use of journalists from political and religious beats means that the scientific details of the ES cell debate get leveled out and that each side is treated as having equivalent amounts of evidence to support their point of view (Taylor & Condit, 1988). Because the journalistic coverage focuses on political issues first, it treats the debate as a tit-for-tat, two-sided argument. Not only does this eliminate any clear evidentiary reason to support one side more than the other, it contributes to a Manichean idiom by creating the appearance of two opposing forces with no common ground or means of adjudicating between them. The only way to resolve the issue is to defeat the opposing side and impose one's point of view on the nation through political maneuvering.

Second, alongside the political focus of most of the coverage, the use of abortion as scene limits the range of ethical issues that can be effectively addressed. A report from the Institute of Medicine's National Research Council (2002) and a report from The President's Council on Bioethics (2004) both identified several ethical issues surrounding ES cell research: These included concerns about the role of the federal government in scientific research, concerns about overselling the promise of ES cell research to produce cures, concerns about how the need for raw materials to create new stem cells will adversely impact women's health, and concerns about access to what might be an expensive medical procedure should ES cells produce cures. Not only does the journalistic focus on abortion limit the range of ethical issues considered, it also shapes audience expectations that a Manichean idiom will characterize the opposition. If abortion is the stage, then the figures on that stage will be expected to act in ways that comport with it. Religious idioms will be expected, and if opponents make arguments or provide definitions using another idiom, the difference between the idiom expected and the idiom used can complicate attempts at persuasion.

Third, such a scene fails to encompass and make sense of the actions within the debate. If the scene of abortion did successfully contain the action of the ES cell debate, then knowing a person's stand on abortion would mean knowing their stand on ES cell research, but some pro-life individuals support ES cell research. These situations do not fit neatly into a scene understood purely in terms of abortion.

Many journalistic uses of abortion overlook this break with the expectations inherent in scene, but 10 of the 28 television news segments and 3 of the 35 newspaper articles that place the debate in the context of abortion address the fact that some pro-life politicians support ES cell research. The journalistic coverage of individuals like Health and Human Services (HHS) secretary Tommy Thompson and Sens. Bill Frist (R–TN) and Orrin Hatch (R–UT) uses a rhetorical *paradox* that ultimately contains this break from the expected pro-life position. Paradoxes present an apparent contradiction, such as a pro-life figure supporting a type of research condemned by most opponents of abortion, which evokes some measure of truth. Its use here adds an element of greater controversy to the story, while reinforcing the link between ES cell research and ethical issues involving the beginning of life.

Most stories that report on pro-life politicians supporting the research emphasize the moral component of their support. A CNN report succinctly notes, "The ethics are as complex as the politics. Some of the most adamant anti-abortion members of Congress are for embryonic stem cell research" ("Stem Cell Research," 2001). In an ABC story on religious attitudes toward ES cell research, reporter Terry Moran says, "But polls show that Catholics are divided over this issue, as they don't always follow the Pope's teaching on other subjects" ("President Bush Meets," 2001). The split in the pro-life camp, into which the national media group all Catholics, becomes a key point in television news coverage on the night of the president's decision. CBS describes Sen. Bill Frist this way: "A staunch opponent of abortion, Frist, like many other Senate conservatives, believes stem cell research is a right-to-life issue for people suffering terminal illness" ("President Bush Supports," 2001). CNN's political commentator Jeff Greenfield reminds viewers, "You know, one thing that's very important to remember is that this is not a case in which the President is taking on an entire constituency. The pro-life movement is split. I won't say it's down the middle, but it's split all over the place on this issue, where some of the more prominent pro-life members of the House and Senate have come out for stem cell research"

("President Bush Makes Decision," 2001). An emphasis is made on the splits and differences in the pro-life movement. A few individuals, like Greenfield, emphasize the political nature of the split—that the divisions in the group alter the dynamics of political decision making and give President Bush room to maneuver in crafting a policy—but most stories emphasize the moral and ethical quality of this divide. Interestingly, only television news stories address this split in the pro-life movement with any detail. Only three newspaper articles in the sample discuss this split, and little detail is provided. *The Omaha World Herald's* story titled "Stem-cell Debate Picks Up" (Olson, 2000e) simply states, "There are anti-abortion politicians who favor embryonic stem-cell research." Similarly sparse prose appears in *The Boston Globe:* "Some fervently antiabortion legislators have publicly supported embryonic stem cell work" (Mishra, 2001a). The most detail comes in *The Milwaukee Journal Sentinel,* in part because former Wisconsin governor Tommy Thompson plays a central role in the story being reported: "It is widely assumed that Thompson is a leader of the pro-funding camp in the White House, even though the cabinet secretary is 'pro-life' and many anti-abortion leaders passionately oppose using public funds for the research" (Gilbert & Skiba, 2001).

The difference in the coverage of the split in the pro-life movement might be a result of different considerations for each medium. Television news must encapsulate a story in an easily understandable format. Using abortion as the scene for the ES cell debate does that. The split in the constituency adds another element of controversy to the issue, allowing television news to further hype the story to increase viewers. While newspapers likewise make use of controversy, they also have a greater amount of space to address a variety of issues related to the ES cell debate that do not directly relate to abortion. This is one possible reason that abortion does not appear in newspaper coverage of the debate as often.

In addition to increasing the controversy connected to the story and thus increasing its potential to draw viewers and readers, the use of paradox performs four other important functions. First, it provides a more accurate depiction of the ES cell debate than the straightforward use of abortion to set the scene: straightforward uses of abortion do not address the splits in the pro-life movement. Second, the portrayal of these pro-life supporters of ES cell research points to a more nuanced ethical debate. While the details of how supporting ES cell research constitutes a pro-life position do not appear in these television reports, reporting this allows the audience to consider these possibilities on their own.[3] Third, this continues to limit the ethical and political debate to issues related to abortion. While the paradox implies a break with the abortion scene, it maintains the Manichean idiom: The apparent contradiction of the paradox allows for some added complexity in religious views of embryonic life, but those truths are still contained by the abortion scene and the Manichean idiom that develops from it. Fourth, the depiction of pro-life, pro–ES cell senators and representatives increases the difficulty for pro-life, anti–ES cell politicians who advocate for a ban on the research, especially in front of their legislative colleagues who support it. Those politicians must distance themselves from abortion as the scene for understanding the debate, while still using the Manichean idiom and the argumentative resources of the abortion debate to invent their anti–ES cell arguments.

Political Disavowals of Abortion as Scene

Journalists have made abortion the scene from which to understand the ES cell debate, but that effort has been complicated by the fact that some vociferous opponents of abortion support ES cell research. For example, in a July 2001 hearing, Senator Hatch declares, "Let me be absolutely clear. I hold strong pro-life, pro-family values and strongly oppose abortion. I conclude that support of embryonic stem cell research is consistent with and advances pro-life and pro-family values" (*Stem Cells, 2001,* 2001, p. 11). Because of statements like this from prominent and powerful pro-life politicians, opponents who would use the rhetorical resources of the abortion debate against ES cell research must undo the perception of ES cell research and abortion as coterminous. Nigel Cameron from the Centre for Bioethics and Public Policy argues, "I do believe that in this discussion we are in danger of losing sight of the middle ground in the assessment of the early embryo. That is to say, this is not a rerun of *Roe.* This is not essentially a debate about the implications of our stance on the abortion issue" (*Stem Cells, 2001,* 2001, p. 95). Senator Sam Brownback (R-KS) makes a similar remark: "Now, despite some similarities, this debate is not about abortion, and I don't think it should be confused with that debate" (*Cloning, 2001,* 2001, p. 5). Both Cameron and Brownback try to distance opposition to ES cell research from the abortion debate, while still employing rhetorical strategies central to pro-life rhetoric later in their testimony. While opposition to abortion and ES cell research might appear to be the same, they argue, the two issues are distinct.

Pro-life opponents of ES cell research also use this distinction in order to create the appearance of a bipartisan opposition to ES cell research. Usually this occurs during discussions of therapeutic cloning—a process for obtaining stem cells that are genetically identical to a person and would not be rejected by their bodies following a tissue or organ transplant. Rep. Dave Weldon (R-FL) argues,

Some people have tried to portray this as a pro-life/pro-choice type of debate. While there may be some people who may view it in that context, if you actually look at what went on in the House, it pretty much transcended that, in that there were a lot of people who were very pro-choice in their outlook, some of whom had a 100-percent approval from various groups like NARAL [National Association for the Repeal of Abortion Laws, now called NARAL Pro-Choice America], who voted for the ban. . . . I say all this to just emphasize that this is not an abortion debate. (*Dangers of Cloning,* 2002)

Weldon makes this argument in order to tie his own objections to therapeutic cloning and ES cell research to the objections from some feminist and environmental groups about the burdens placed on women by biomedical technology, which appear in testimony from 2002.[4] While the objections to ES cell research from liberal groups almost never appear in the journalistic coverage of the issue, Weldon tries to link his pro-life-based concerns about cloning and ES cell research to the concerns of environmentalist and feminist speakers concerned about the impact of biotechnology on women's health.

Pro-life opponents of ES cell research must decouple their objections to ES cell research from the debates about abortion, and they try to present the objections of progressive groups as identical to their own. They do so for two reasons. First, ES cell research challenges the unity of the pro-life coalition: Prominent members of that group support ES cell research, making a unified message on this issue difficult at best. Second, by decoupling ES cell research and abortion, opponents try to establish grounds for using a scientistic idiom. If they can use a scientistic idiom, they can present their concerns about the embryo as real definitions with scientific backing in the same way that definitions of ES cells as potential cures for devastating illness are presented. This helps mitigate against views of the debate as a contest between "scientific fact" and "religious opinions." Yet, this approach is problematic for pro-life rhetors. First, decoupling the debate from abortion, while simultaneously using anti-abortion rhetoric as the basis for their argument, fails to address the divide between religious basis for much pro-life rhetoric and a scientistic idiom, which originally prompted the move to separate abortion and ES cell research. Second, the claims for a bipartisan set of objections are rejected by the progressive speakers, especially Judy Norsigian of the Boston Women's Health Book Collective, who says, "At the outset, let me make clear that my organization and many of our colleagues in the women's health and reproductive rights movements support embryonic stem cell research, but we also believe that a moratorium on all human embryo cloning is necessary at this point in time" (*Dangers of Cloning,* 2002, p. 24). Decoupling the objections to ES cell research from abortion does not help opponents recruit others to their cause nor does it clarify the political and ethical issues at hand in the debate. The scene of abortion remains a constant as opponents use the rhetoric of the pro-life movement to make their case against ES cell research.

Abortion and Invention: Using Pro-life Rhetoric against ES Cell Research

While journalists use the abortion debate as a scene that makes the ES cell debate intelligible, the arguments and rhetorical strategies used in abortion also act as a source for the *invention* of arguments by definition in the ES cell debate. Opponents of ES cell research turn to familiar pro-life strategies and use the figure of the public fetus—the rhetorical construction of the fetus as an autonomous person separate from its mother (Petchesky, 1990)—to give their claims persuasive power. This image of fetal life has been a metonym for all the stages of human development from conception to birth, and although it stands for *all* developing life, its symbolic power derives from images of late-pregnancy fetuses that easily fit visual conventions for depicting people (Condit, 1990). It is a key strategy of pro-life rhetoric, and while pro-life rhetoric appears purely spiritual or religious in basis, the public fetus has scientistic elements insofar as it takes visual and discursive elements from science, like images of a fetus, and incorporates them into a public vocabulary. Furthermore, as I will show below, its use in the ES cell debate moves beyond the ambit of a scientistic idiom to become a form of "biorhetoric," a strategy by which moral and political positions are interwoven with apparently neutral statements of biological "fact" (Lyne, 1990). In congressional discourse, opponents ground the extension of the public fetus to the embryo primarily in biology instead of religious or spiritual concerns, thus using the trappings of biology to lend certitude to the moral and social implications of the public fetus. To borrow Lyne's language (which he in turn borrowed from David Hume), this argument by definition simultaneously defines what *is* and derives from it an *ought*. These arguments establish a fact and derive a moral judgment from it.

The application of the public fetus to the ES cell debate has been made problematic not only because prominent pro-life politicians support ES cell research but also because the technological and cultural practices that made the public fetus so powerful in the abortion debate undermine its rhetorical power vis-à-vis the ES cell debate. This means that claims for the "personhood" of the embryo—claims for its status as a living human being deserving protection equal to the protection granted those already born—cannot be made unproblematically. Opponents try explicitly to extend the reach of the public fetus by using the rhetorical figure of *incrementum* to connect the public fetus to earlier, embryonic stages of life. While journalistic reporting transfers claims from the abortion debate to the ES cell debate, political discourse about ES cell research intensifies the biorhetorical and scientistic elements of the debate, increasing the importance of scientific authority in making the case for or against ES cell research. After discussing the rhetoric of the public fetus, the remainder of this chapter will examine the opponents' attempts to define the embryo as the key point of moral objection to ES cell research.

"Fetus" and "Embryo"

In addition to being a biological entity, the fetus has a "public" life outside of the womb (Petchesky, 1990). The "public fetus" is a rhetorical figure that animates debates about abortion. It stands for a being that has rights independent of others, especially its mother, and it has become "a seemingly permanent fixture on the popular cultural scene" (Casper, 1998, p. 16).[5] The public fetus combines a scientistic idiom and biorhetoric and creates a real definition which lends certitude to the moral and social implications drawn from it. The argument goes that the public fetus is a rights-bearing individual *because* science has shown it to be so. In this section, I will outline the discursive and visual elements that constitute the rhetorical figure of the public fetus and then highlight scientific-cultural practices that alter the symbol's persuasive power.

As Monica Casper (1998) notes, debates about abortion are "framed around static biological definitions of personhood and life, embodied in the compelling image of the tiny homunculus" (p. 17). This homunculus—this public image of developing life—exists because of a combination of discursive and visual rhetoric. The primary discursive strategy consists of a series of terms that slowly extends personhood from actual, born people to developing humans. As Schiappa (2003) notes, despite their failure in *Roe v. Wade*, "anti-abortion advocates often defend the linkage *fetus = live human being = person*" (p. 97). This series is used to extend the definition of person, as an individual protected by the Fourteenth Amendment of the Constitution, to fetal life, and it represents the primary discursive component of the public fetus.

The extension of individual rights has focused on the *fetus*. Yet, the debate surrounding ES cell research focuses on the *embryo*. Discussion in the public sphere has focused on the fetus instead of the embryo because the two terms are treated as equivalent. Through a metonymic reduction, all stages of developing life become the "unborn": "the wide variety of beings that constitute developing unborn human life-forms—the blastocyst, embryo, fetus, viable baby— were reduced to a single entity through the creation of a single vision of the 'unborn baby'" (Condit, 1990, p. 82). The public fetus stands for all developing life. Furthermore, this metonymy provides the basis for the public fetus's visual element: The third-trimester fetus becomes the public image representing all developing human life. Images of other stages of development would not have worked: "We do not see images of blastocysts or piglike fetuses, nor do we see malformed fetuses held up as emblems of the individual. . . . We usually see a perfect, baby-like fetus of several months" (Stormer, 2000, p. 130). The visual similarity between the late-stage fetus and fully developed humans is central to the persuasive power of the public fetus. Earlier forms of life, such as blastocysts (one of the earliest stages of embryonic life) that are used in ES cell research, do not appear human. This makes it difficult to create the sense of identification that is a key component of the public fetus.

The visual component of the public fetus is made possible in part because of specific technological and cultural practices. The first practice is fetal surgery, in which surgeons temporarily remove a fetus from the womb, operate on it, and replace it in the hopes that it will be carried to term and be healthy (Casper, 1998; Williams, Alderson, & Farsides, 2001). This practice has helped define the fetus as a patient with rights and legal interests distinct from its pregnant mother, and this status as a patient has been the basis for portraying the mother and fetus as having opposing interests (Casper, 1998; Hartouni, 1997; Oaks, 2000).[6]

Techniques of fetal imaging, from photographs to the ultrasound image, have also shaped contemporary understandings of the public fetus. Not only does this technology provide raw images of a fetus, but the construction and framing of these images help shape the visual component of the public fetus by, often literally, erasing the mother from the pictures (Casper, 1998; Duden, 1993; Petchesky, 1990; Stabile, 1994; Stormer, 2000). Stormer describes the standard image: It consists of "a darkened or neutral background broken by the spherical border of the amniotic sac, occasionally with some placental mass attached or without any sac at all. The fetus rests serenely, alone, sometimes with its thumb in its mouth. As a photograph the image is often backlit to add a translucent, ethereal quality to the fetus" (p. 128). Stormer argues that visual schemes of individualism frame this image to create a "prenatal space" wherein the fetus is the only actor, the only person: "The womb is purified by the erasure of the woman, as well as the doctor, family, community and so forth" (p. 129).

While fetal surgery and fetal imaging help create and reinforce the power of the public fetus, the effect of in vitro fertilization (IVF) technology has been ambivalent. According to Patricia Spallone (1989), "On the one hand, IVF practitioners assure everyone that they have due respect for embryos. On the other hand, these same IVF practitioners must handle and inevitably destroy or discard human embryos" (p. 21).[7] IVF produces embryos in order to fulfill the desire of infertile couples to have children, but the technology produces embryos in surplus of a couple's needs. This raises the issue of "spare" or "orphan embryos" (Franklin, 1999; Hartouni, 1997). The existence of these embryos raises concerns about legal status, guardianship, and even property rights: "Whose property were they, what was their status, the nature of their relationship to each other and their 'genetic sponsors,' the extent of their claims? Should they be thawed and flushed, used for experimentation, or 'put up for adoption'?" (Hartouni, 1997, p. 28). IVF raises questions about the storage of embryos, their destruction, their use in research, and the possibility of "embryo adoption." While Great Britain has a set of laws dealing with the disposition of spare embryos (Franklin, 1999), the United States has no such framework. In fact, a moratorium on federally funded research on IVF existed until 1993 because some people feared the impact that IVF research would have on our understanding of the unborn (Fletcher, 2001).

Other medical developments have produced views of the fetus that run counter to the public fetus. While some elements of medical science treat the fetus and embryo as "person" or "patient," other elements treat both as "prime work objects" (Casper, 1998, p. 214). Health-care workers—ranging from midwives to obstetricians, genetic counselors to pediatricians—view developing human lives as "nobody" or a commodity as often as they view them as patients or persons (Williams et al., 2001). A similar range of views exists in federal law and practice: *Roe v. Wade* rejected the arguments about the personhood of fetuses (Schiappa, 2003), but the Centers for Disease Control and Prevention collects information about "fetal death" for developing humans after 20 weeks of gestation (Centers for Disease Control, 2004).[8] Since the development of IVF in the mid-1970s, the U.S. government has debated the issue of fetal and embryonic tissue research. As part of the conservative trend in politics since the 1980s, the federal government has progressively restricted research on developing humans, starting with a ban on federal funding of fetal research in 1984 and a ban on embryonic research in 1996 (Fletcher, 2001).

While the public fetus is central to debates about reproductive issues, its symbolic power is potentially limited by its dependency on images of late-term fetuses. While these images provide a resource for identification—late-term fetuses appear human—this identification, and the persuasive power that accompanies it, might not be activated when discussing earlier stages of developing life that do not appear human. Even blanket statements that "life begins at conception" depend in part on the public fetus for their persuasive force, and when the power of the public fetus is limited, the space is opened to separate the "fetus" and the "embryo" as different in kind, not merely different in degree. This difference between the two terms helps shape debates about ES cell research. Because the "embryo" used in ES cell research is not noticeably human, the power of the public fetus is not automatically activated. This might help explain, in part, why some staunchly pro-life senators, like Orrin Hatch (R-UT) and Bill Frist (R-TN), support funding for ES cell research. Since the power of the public fetus is not automatically activated, opponents of ES cell research must elaborate on the arguments grounded in the public fetus, while proponents try to confound that elaboration and treat embryos as qualitatively different from fetuses. This argument occurs in two parts. First, opponents try to argue that ES cells *are* embryos, while proponents separate the two. This debate occurs because the Dickey Amendment, first passed in 1995 and attached to all subsequent appropriations bills funding the National Institutes of Health, bans all federal funding of embryo research: If ES cells are embryos, then the U.S. government cannot fund ES cell research. Second, opponents of ES cell research try to extend the rhetorical reach of the public fetus to the earliest forms of human life.

Separating Stem Cells and Embryos

The first stage of the debate about ES cells and embryos focused on issues of identity: Opponents of ES cell research tried to define ES cells as embryos, while proponents defined ES cells and embryos as qualitatively different entities. This debate begins with a presumption of identity: Since a ban on embryonic research was in place, any research associated with embryos was suspect. Opponents tried to cement that identity, and proponents had to separate the two categories in order to obtain federal funding for this research. Senator Tom Harkin (D-IA) clearly states the issue at the beginning of the first hearing on ES cells: "The key question that I hope will be addressed today is whether under current law scientists can use Dr. Thomson's stem cells for federally funded research. These stem cells do not have the capacity to become a human being, and, therefore, it is my belief, my opinion, that they do not fall under the ban on human embryo research" (*Stem Cell Research,* 1999, p. 3). In order for research to go forward, ES cells must not fall under the ban on human embryo research. In framing the issue, Harkin, a supporter of ES cell research, also makes the key definitional move separating ES cells and embryos—ES cells cannot lead to the development of a human being.

The scientists, who were the first group to testify in the hearing, reiterate Harkin's claim. NIH director Dr. Harold Varmus claims that embryonic stem and germ cells are not like embryos since they cannot form the type of cells an embryo needs to implant in the uterus:

Unlike the fertilized egg, or the early embryo, or the intact blastocyst, neither the disaggregated inner cell mass nor the pluripotent stem cells derived from it (nor the pluripotent stem cells derived from fetal germ cells) will produce a human being even if returned to a woman's uterus. These cells do not have the potential to form a human being, because they do not have the capacity to give rise to the cells of the placenta or other extraembryonic tissues necessary for implantation, nor can they support fetal development in the uterus. (*Stem Cell Research,* 1999, pp.8–9)

Varmus enumerates a variety of cell types that ES cells are incapable of producing. Since all these cells are necessary for an embryo to implant in the uterus and develop, Varmus's testimony separates ES cells from the continuum of human development.

Following Varmus's elaborate separation of ES cells from embryos, the scientists who testify after him do not use the same amount of rhetorical labor in defining ES cells as distinct from embryos. Some simply assert that ES cells and embryos are not the same thing. For example, Dr. John Gearhart says, "It is important to note that while these cells have the capacity to form a variety of cell types, they cannot form embryos" (p. 13). Dr. James Thomson makes the same claim with more detail: "Human ES cell lines are not the equivalent of an intact human embryo. If a clump of ES cells was transferred to a woman's uterus, the ES cells would not implant and would not form a viable fetus" (*Stem Cell Research,* 1999, p. 18). Thomson asserts that ES cells are not like an embryo: They can form many cell types, but they cannot develop into a full grown human. Thomson and Gearhart do not fully develop this argument for two reasons. They follow Varmus who provided more detail in response to this concern, and their status as the scientists who originally isolated ES and embryonic germ (EG) cells allows them to make the assertion without fully developing it.

Others rhetors in this hearing use scientific expertise or practice to define ES cells and embryos as qualitatively different and reaffirm that ES cell research is eligible for federal funding. Dr. Michael West bases his claim that ES cells are not embryos on science's collective experience with ES cells from animals: "If they are, for instance, grown in a laboratory dish or transplanted into a uterus, they will not form a human being. They have never been observed to form a complete animal using the animal equivalent of these cells" (*Stem Cell Research,* 1999, p. 30). Previous work on animal stem cells, West argues, has shown that ES cells do not lead to a fully developed organism, whether that organism is an animal or a human being. Dr. Thomas Okarma's testimony continues the trend in the previous testimonies to identify ES cells as only a part of the embryo, but he emphasizes the intervention of scientists as another reason to separate the two. He implies that scientific intervention creates the division between embryonic stem cells and embryos: "My view is that these cells are clearly not organisms. They are highly derived by a laboratory process that took years to develop and in fact, as we have said, are not the cellular equivalent of an embryo. Were these cells to be implanted, they would not form a conceptus nor develop" (*Stem Cell Research,* 1999, p. 71). According to Okarma, ES cells are not embryos since they are synthetic, the end result of a laboratory process, and embryos are natural, the end result of sexual activity. Because of this, the cells would not develop into a person. Both testimonies reiterate the position that embryonic stem cells are not capable of forming a whole person; therefore they are not embryos, which *are* capable of producing the whole human.

The arguments employed by Varmus, Gearhart, Thomson, West, and Okarma are reiterated throughout this stage of the debate. While testifying about the health implications of stem cell research, Dr. Douglas Melton asserts, "Stem cells have the potential to develop into any tissue or organ in the body and yet cannot develop into a full human being" (*Stem Cell Research,* 1999, p. 101). Dr. Lawrence Goldstein's argument in April 2000, mimics Dr. West's claims from the first hearing: "Research work over the past 20 years using mouse embryonic stem cells has demonstrated that these cells by themselves cannot form an adult organism, but they can differentiate into an adult cell type" (*Stem Cell Research, part 3,* 2000, p. 43). By the time Dr. Richard Hynes baldly states that ES cells are not embryos in September 2000, he does not need evidence to support the assertion because legal rulings and NIH guidelines for ES cell research have transformed the claim from assertion to legally accepted fact (*Stem Cell Research, part 3,* 2000, p. 84).

Opponents try to reinforce the position that ES cells are embryos. Richard Doerflinger, a spokesman for the United States Conference of Catholic Bishops, tries to define ES and EG cells as embryos during testimony on ES cell research in December 1998, and January 1999. His attack focuses primarily on research in Dr. Gearhart's lab:

> Are the primordial germ cells obtained from abortion victims being used to create human embryos, which are then destroyed or suppressed to provide tissue? . . . There is some ambiguity in current reports of the new research, because the researchers speak of collecting "embryoid bodies" from these cultures and finding "derivatives of all three embryonic germ layers" in the culture. They add that some of these bodies form "complex structures closely resembling an embryo during early development" and that

they "appear to recapitulate the normal developmental processes of early embryonic stages and promote the cell-cell interaction required for cell differentiation." (*Stem Cell Research,* 1999, pp. 47–48)

While quoting the research report announcing the isolation of embryonic germ cells (i.e., Shamblott et al., 1998), Doerflinger does three things. First, he ties the ES cell debate back to the abortion debate with his reference to "abortion victims." This is somewhat effective in this case because he focuses on EG cells that are isolated from fetuses in the second trimester of development, instead of the 14-day-old blastocysts that produce ES cells. Second, he employs the rhetorical figure of *polyptoton,* the similarity and repetition of parts of words (Fahnestock, 1999), to establish an identity between the EG cells and embryos. Doerflinger emphasizes the similarity of "embryoid" to "embryo" to imply that embryoid bodies are embryos.[9] Third, he defines cells as simple, and embryos as complex. Since Gearhart's cells form complex structures, it is questionable, for Doerflinger, whether these samples are "only cells."

Later in the hearing, Doerflinger remarks, "So I think that it is an open question with regard to Dr. Gearhart's experiment whether in the course of this experiment he is actually creating some early embryos in the culture. I think the answer is no, but I do not know, and I do not know that anyone knows" (*Stem Cell Research,* 1999, p. 71). While he admits his lack of knowledge about the research, he also argues that no one else knows the answers to the questions he raises, thus implying that scientists lack the grounds to claim that ES and EG cells are not embryos. In January 1999, Doerflinger offers a modification of his original conclusion: "A stem cell is not an organism, but the possibility must be explored that groups of stem cells may recongregate in some of this research to form an entity that is, however briefly, a living organism" (p. 132). Here, Doerflinger concedes the point that stem cells are not organisms, and therefore not embryos. Yet, he argues that ES cells have the power to "recongregate" and become an embryo: The *telos* of embryonic development is so great, that it could reassert itself.

The claim that ES cells can become embryos is repeated by two other opponents of this research. Dr. David Prentice also argues that embryonic stem cells can form embryos:

The publications regarding human or primate embryonic stem cells and their derivation note that, unlike [mouse] embryonic stem cells, human and primate embryonic stem cells can form not only tissues that become part of the human body, but also trophoblast tissue . . . . Now, reformation of this tissue layer in cultures of embryonic stem cells could lead to reformation of complete human embryos in culture, able to survive if implanted into a womb. (*Stem Cell Research, part 3,* 2000, pp. 62–63)

The prepared testimony for the Center for Bioethics and Human Dignity says, "Some evidence suggests that stem cells cultured in the laboratory may have a tendency to recongregate and form an aggregate of cells capable of beginning to develop as an embryo" (*Opportunities and Advancements,* 2001, p. 392). The respective testimonies of Prentice and the Center reiterate Doerflinger's claim: The ability to form complex structures and cell types implies the beginning of a human life.

Proponents and opponents ground their arguments in biological processes, but the attempt by opponents to define embryonic stem cells as embryos does not succeed. This argument blurs the line between a scientistic idiom and science. It goes beyond the use of scientific language to make a specific scientific argument about the biological nature of ES cells for which there was no evidence. The scientific literature on human ES cells extant during the period this argument was made did not provide any evidence to support claims that stem cells could recongregate into embryos. Also, none of the individuals making these claims had worked with ES cells in the laboratory. This includes Prentice, who was the only person with a medical or scientific background to make the claim. Since the argument has moved onto scientific ground, the situation favors the proponents of ES cell research who are predominantly scientists, many of whom have experience with ES cells, and who state their position with a high degree of certitude. Opponents of the research are at a disadvantage making this claim. Most likely, they were aware of this, as evidenced by the tentative and often convoluted phrasing of this argument.

The weakness of these arguments is reflected in the sparse journalistic coverage this aspect of the ES cell debate received. ABC News reports on the Dickey Amendment and how it bars the federal government from supporting ES cell research: "Congress has barred federal funding for research involving human embryos on the grounds that embryos are already human beings. That puts the dream of creating things like new spinal cords for paraplegics even farther away" ("Enormous Scientific Breakthrough," 1998). An early report on ES cell research in *The Washington Post* concedes that ambiguity exists about the nature of stem cells and embryos: "In the new biology, the distinction between embryo cells and other cells has blurred" (Weiss, 1998). The article later paraphrases Michael West: "It is not clear whether stem cells are technically embryos or not, especially after they have been growing and multiplying in a lab dish for months" (Weiss, 1998). While the article acknowledges uncertainty about ES cells and their status as embryos, the balance of the article implies that ES cells are not embryos. By January of 1999, *The Milwaukee Journal Sentinel* reports on a legal opinion from the Department of Health and Human Services that "a 1994 [*sic*] congressional ban on using federal money for human embryo research did not apply to stem cells 'because such cells are not an embryo' and cannot develop into a human being" (Marchione, 1999; see also Schmickle, 1999a). By May 1999, Cleveland's *Plain Dealer* simply states, "Researchers emphasize that the inner cell mass alone cannot produce a viable embryo" (Haybron, 1999). The argument that ES cells are embryos does not have a lot of power: It shifts the argument from the scientistic idiom of the public sphere to technical grounds and scientific expertise, which puts opponents at a disadvantage, and it does not receive significant media attention. Because of this, opponents turn to more familiar arguments from the abortion debate to argue that ES cell extraction is the murder of a developing human life.

Extending Personhood to the Embryo

After arguments that ES cells were actually fetuses failed to stop federal funding and congressional consideration of this research, opponents began to deploy arguments familiar from debates about abortion. Opponents of ES research must make the embryo a person and the derivation of ES cells its murder. Pro-life abortion rhetoric employs a metonymic reduction of all developing life to the "fetus." Claims such as "life begins at conception" are the ultimate metonymy, eliminating all differences between the various stages of life. But in the ES cell debate, opponents must explicitly *extend* the definition of personhood from fully developed humans and the fetus down the chain of developmental forms to the embryo and the blastocyst. Extension of definitions is a recurring use for rhetorical figures that form a series (Fahnestock, 1999). Pro-life rhetoric has already created the series *fetus = live human being = person* that only requires extension to other stages of developing human life. This extension appears in both news coverage of the debate and political discourse, but some key differences exist. Media coverage emphasizes the moral component of the objections to ES cell research, reinforcing the dichotomy between science and religion/morality that is central to a Manichean idiom. While political arguments use many of the same strategies, they intensify the biorhetorical elements of pro-life rhetoric. Opponents ground extensions of the public fetus and its rhetorical potential to the embryo primarily in biology instead of religious or spiritual concerns.

Defining Objections to ES Cell Research as Moral or Religious

Because they use abortion as the grounds for rendering the ES cell debate intelligible, news media describe the opposition to ES cell research only as moral or religious. A *Tampa Tribune* article observes that a government commission's support of ES cell research "roused those who believe embryonic research is immoral, those who believe that the destruction of an embryo amounts to the taking of a human life" ("Dealing with Hard Ethical Questions," 2000). *The New York Times* notes, "But such cells are at the center of an ethical controversy, with opponents saying it is immoral to use embryos for medical purposes" (Pollack, 2000). *The St. Louis Post-Dispatch* makes a similar observation: "Opponents say such research is morally wrong because it requires the destruction of embryos— which they say are human lives—in the process" (Hesman, 2001b). Often, the news coverage uses direct quotes from opponents to establish the moral basis for their objections. *The Omaha World Herald's* coverage of the Clinton administration's guidelines for funding ES cell research paraphrased Sister Renee Mirkes, a Catholic nun on the University of Nebraska's bioethics committee: "She said they give the federal government the luxury of supporting embryonic stem-cell research while ignoring the more ethically challenging process of how those stem cells are obtained" (Olson, 2000c). CNN interviewed National Right to Life executive director David O'Steen, who argued, "It's morally, ethically *and* scientifically wrong to use tax funds to pay to deliberately kill human embryos for research purposes" ("Landmark in Embryo Research," 2001). A CBS news segment in July 2001 included an interview with Richard Doerflinger: "We have, you know, an absolute view that the ends don't justify the means, that exploiting or destroying innocent life at any stage is not justified by the consequences" ("Controversy Brewing," 2001). An ABC news report on the eve of Bush's ES cell research decision includes remarks from the Family Research Council's Ken Connor: "If the federal government embraces embryonic stem cell research, what that means is we'll have embraced a new and very dangerous medical ethic" ("Possibility for Private Funding," 2001).

The news coverage also highlights the religious component of these objections by emphasizing the role of the Catholic Church in leading opposition to ES cell research. While a handful of articles identify "religious conservatives" as the key group opposing ES cell research ("President Bush Supports," 2001; Kiely, 2001b; Stolberg, 2001b), many articles narrow the focus to the Catholic Church itself. In June 2001, *The New York Times* names three groups as the bulk of the opposition to ES cell research: "Anti-abortion groups, conservatives and the Roman Catholic Church object on moral grounds to using stem cells extracted from embryos, even those at fertility clinics that might otherwise be discarded" (Pear, 2001). In the week prior to President Bush's decision on ES cell research, *The Houston Chronicle* extensively quotes the objections of Houston's bishop, Joseph Fiorenza, to ES cell research (Dooley, 2001). *USA Today* most frequently identifies the Catholic Church as a bulwark of the opposition. One article points to it as the leader of the opposition: "Opponents led by the Catholic

Church believe destroying embryos for research is against the sanctity of life" (Friend, 2001f). This claim is repeated in an article printed shortly before the president's decision in August 2001 (Friend, 2001e). The lead of the article discussing ethical concerns about ES cell research contrasts Catholic and Jewish attitudes toward the research and treats them as exemplars of the gap between opponents and supporters of the research (Friend, 2001b). Around this time, the role of the Catholic Church in leading opponents of ES cell research is cemented by news coverage of President Bush's visit to the Vatican near the end of July 2001. ABC, CBS, CNN, and NBC all reported on the visit, and all of them aired in part John Paul II's declaration that ES cell research violates human dignity ("George Bush Visits," 2001; "President Bush Discusses," 2001; "President Bush Meets," 2001; "President Bush Receives," 2001). NBC's Brian Williams highlighted the importance of this encounter: "They are, arguably, the two most powerful men in the world: the American President, George W. Bush, and Pope John Paul II. On the agenda on their meeting today was what is rapidly becoming one of the most emotional, polarizing and controversial issues of our time: the use of cells from human embryos for research" ("George Bush Visits," 2001). All of these statements highlight the religious component of objections to ES cell research, and these statements further narrow the scope of "religious objections" to "Catholic objections." The focus on Catholic objections represents a problematic use of *synecdoche:* It reduces religion to a single emblematic religious group, and while that group is one of the largest Christian denominations in the United States and plays a prominent role in the pro-life and anti–ES cell movement, this reduction deflects attention away from other prominent groups and the loose-knit nature of the opposition to ES cell research. This focus on religious objections generally and Catholic objections specifically helps cast the debate as a fight between science and religion. Traditionally, uses of a Manichean idiom have forced the Catholic Church to represent religion in depictions of deep-seated conflict between science and religion (Lessl, 1999, 2007). Using the Catholic Church to stand in for all religious opposition to ES cell research reflects and extends the role it plays in other manifestations of the Manichean idiom.

Extending Personhood in the News

In addition to signaling the moral and religious nature of the opposition, news media often present some of the attempts by opponents to extend the public fetus to the earliest stages of embryonic human life. Many news reports present the extension of the public fetus and the status of person as a simple declaration. *The St. Louis Post-Dispatch* reports that opponents "say such research destroys embryos, which they consider human life" (Hesman, 2000). Many newspapers use a variation of *USA Today's* statement that "some regard this as taking a life" (Vergano, 2001a).[10] Some report opponents' view of ES cell research as an exchange of one human life for another. *The Omaha World Herald* reports, "Opponents of embryonic research consider it taking a life to save a life" (Olson, 2001). An NBC news story includes the remarks of New York Medical College's Dr. Daniel Sulmasy, who says, "You're using somebody else—another human being, another human life—as a pure means of helping yourself, and that's fundamentally morally wrong" ("Debate over Stem Cell Research," 2001).[11] This form of the opposition argument defines embryos as human lives treated as the means to a medical end.

Additionally, one finds a use of emotional language to describe the derivation of ES cells from embryos. Most often, news media use the word "destruction" to describe the derivation of ES cells. For example, *The New York Times* reports, "Abortion opponents object to the fact that embryonic stem cells are derived by destroying embryos" (Wade, 2001c). The use of "destruction" is ambiguous. While the destruction of people is a terrible thing, we destroy buildings and bacteria without a second thought. The emotional valence of "destruction" depends on one's attitude toward embryos prior to reading the statement: Specifically, are they more like objects or more like people? Other language clearly supports the view of embryos as people. For example, 15 articles use the word "kill" to describe the derivation of ES cells. "An embryo is killed when the pluripotent stem cells are extracted," says an article from *The St. Louis Post-Dispatch* (Hesman, 2001b). Such language assumes a definition of embryos as human beings. Finally, the language of "harvesting" is used multiple times to describe the derivation of ES cells. *The Houston Chronicle* explains that people are concerned for embryos slated for ES cell research because "the harvesting of their stem cells kills them" (Ackerman & Roth, 2001). *The Boston Globe* says, "Because stem cells are harvested from discarded embryos and fetuses, antiabortion activists equate the harvesting to partial-birth abortion" (Mishra, 2001a), and *The Seattle Times* reports that opponents of ES cell research support adult stem cell research "because 'harvesting' adult cells does not ruin embryos" ("Here's What Debate," 2001). "Harvesting" language implies agriculture and defines the derivation of ES cells as a process that treats embryos as a product grown for human use. While not explicitly declaring that embryos are people, the language of harvesting implies that a callous and unfeeling perspective animates the use of embryos and ES cells, a perspective antithetical to commonplace attitudes toward developing human life.

Many of the objections presented in the news media recapitulate parts of the series extending personhood to embryos. Some focus on the legal aspects of personhood. Minneapolis's *Star Tribune* describes the "millions of Americans who see fetuses and the embryos that precede them as the equivalent of a human life—and therefore to be respected and protected under the law" (Schmickle, 1999a). *The Omaha World Herald* interviewed Dr. David Prentice and reported his belief that "an embryo is a human life that should be assigned rights. It is wrong to destroy embryos, he said, even for the good of others" (Olson, 2000e), and an article the next month notes, "Some object because the research . . . requires the destruction of a human embryo, which they consider a human life with civil rights" (Olson, 2000d). In each case, legal rights and protections that pertain to the category "person" become a key quality that opponents apply to embryos. These extensions of legal rights highlight the issues opponents view as central to the debate, although they do not elucidate the connection of "embryos" to "live human beings" that ultimately results in legal rights.

Many individuals who oppose ES cell research use language that does explicitly define embryos as people. A CBS report quotes Cathy Brown of the American Life League, a pro-life group: "We are talking about a human person in his embryonic stage of development, who is going to be destroyed for scientific gain" ("Scientists and Anti-Abortion," 2001). Another CBS story quotes Richard Doerflinger: "We don't think that human life at any stage of development, even at the embryo's stage, should be harvested for cells for research" ("President Bush's Appeal," 2001). Both references to the stages of human development describe the use of embryos as motivated by the desire to advance science, creating the specter of out-of-control science (see Mulkay, 1996).

Others specifically use images of youth and children to emphasize the continuum of human development. *The Milwaukee Journal Sentinel* states that some "view the manipulation of tissue taken from human embryos as no better than killing unborn babies for the sake of science" (Ward, 2000). An article in *The Atlanta Journal-Constitution* uses the following situation to describe the attitude of opponents:

> If you believe . . . that human life begins the moment a sperm penetrates the wall of a human egg, then each of the 5,000 embryos stored in the RBA lab is a human being in its own right, with a soul and all the rights inherent in any other human being. You would no more use these "preborn children" to create spare parts than you would kidnap a child off the street and strip him of his organs. (Bookman, 2001)

According to this perspective, embryos are children yet to be born. A CBS news segment uses a clip from a congressional panel where Sen. Sam Brownback declares, "The principle being denied in this case is the dignity of the young human, effectively making the human embryo equal to mere plant or animal life" ("Influential Senator Bill Frist," 2001). Personhood is extended through depicting embryos as babies and young humans.

Finally, some, especially members of the National Right to Life, use the language of family to encapsulate metaphorically the entire human race and all potential human life. *The Milwaukee Journal Sentinel* quoted the following statement from the National Right to Life: "Members of the human family certainly should not be used for harmful experimentation or destroyed based on their method of creation" (Marchione, 1998). A CBS news segment includes National Right to Life's legislative director, Douglas Johnson, who declares, "This research involves crossing a line and taking the lives of individual members of the human family in order to support scientific research" ("Federal Guidelines for Stem Cell," 2000). The family image creates a family that encompasses all people and all stages of human development, implying that actual, born human beings have the same obligations toward embryos and fetuses that parents, grandparents, and such have to the children within their family.

Statements about the stages of human development and depictions of the embryonic children and a pan-species family supplement declarations that life begins at conception. While some reports emphasize that this position is also a part of Catholic doctrine (Friend, 2001b, 2001f), most treat this as a belief common to many, if not all, opponents of ES cell research, regardless of religious sect. According to *The New York Times,* opponents claim ES cell research "is immoral because they believe that life begins at conception" (Stolberg, 2001c). According to *The Boston Globe,* those holding these beliefs view ES cell research as "murder" (Mishra, 2001a), while *The Atlanta Journal-Constitution* claims the opposition finds the research "morally wrong, no matter the greater good" (Guthrie, 2001). The most extensive description appears in *The Boston Globe* in late August 2001:

> Many believe that life begins the moment the egg and sperm fuse to form the first cell. At this point, they believe, the cell is given a soul, otherwise known as "ensoulment."
>
> By this reasoning, the blastocyst is morally just like a person, endowed with the same basic human rights. To destroy the blastocyst is murder, in their view. And stem cell research, whatever benefit it may have, comes at the expense of this slaughter, they feel. (Mishra, 2001c)

Each statement that life begins at conception uses the public fetus and attempts to create an identity between the potential life of embryos and those lives already born. Further, the moral element of this position is highlighted, especially in the extended quotation from *The Boston Globe* above. Embryos are people not because of a legal decision or because of any biological similarity. Embryos are people because they have souls. The "life" implied in the statement "life begins at conception" can be biological, but the overall trend of the news coverage is to treat said life as a result of having a soul. This stands in contrast to the political debate. While many of the individuals speaking before Congress probably believe in "ensoulment" and object to ES cell research on religious grounds, the emphasis in the political discourse is on biological understandings of life.

Extending Personhood in Political Discourse

Arguments in the news and in politics both depend on the rhetorical figure of the public fetus. The arguments by definition use figurative and emotional language in both areas, but attempts at extending personhood to embryos in political discourse have one major difference. Political arguments extending personhood use a scientistic idiom that emphasizes the biological and scientific bases for their argument rather than morality and religion. This move represents an intensification of the biorhetorical elements of the public fetus. Arguments about the beginning of human life have always blended ethical opinion and scientific fact, but the moral trappings have always remained relatively apparent and constant. In this debate, political arguments increase their reliance on language borrowed from biology and genetics, while expunging more of the moral and religious language. Because religious, pro-life senators support ES cell research, opponents of the research cannot attack proponents as being amoral or against religion. Furthermore, because these debates are intended to shape the policy and legal landscape for scientific research, opponents would have a difficult time making a religious argument because it would be viewed as an imposition on scientific autonomy and as government support for one religious viewpoint, which is not allowed under court interpretations of the First Amendment (Taylor & Condit, 1988; The President's Council on Bioethics, 2004).

In the first hearing on embryonic stem cells in December 1998, Richard Doerflinger grounds the extension of personhood in legal opinion and scientific fact:

> [The Supreme Court] has even allowed states to declare that human life begins at conception, and that it deserves legal protection from that point onward—so long as this principle is not used to place an undue burden on a woman's "right" to choose abortion before viability. . . . Moreover, a scientific consensus now recognizes the status of the early human embryo, and the continuity of human development from the one-celled stage on-

ward, to a greater extent than was true even a few years ago. (*Stem Cell Research,* 1999, p. 46)

In addition to legal grounds for declaring early embryos as people, Doerflinger argues, science also recognizes the "continuity" of life from conception onward. Given the series logic used by ES cell opponents, establishing that something is "human" also established that it is a person who is the bearer of certain rights and deserving of legal protection. Although Doerflinger is present at the hearing as a representative of the Catholic Church, his explicit justification for protecting embryos is scientific and legal, not religious. References to scientific explanations of human development occur in other hearings as well. In his testimony from January 1999, Doerflinger quotes an embryology textbook: "A zygote is the beginning of a new human being" (*Stem Cell Research,* 1999, p. 135n5). The prepared testimony of the Center for Bioethics and Human Dignity notes, "An international scientific consensus now recognizes that human embryos are biologically human beings beginning at fertilization, and acknowledges the physical continuity of human growth and development from the one-cell stage forward" (*Opportunities and Advancements,* 2001, p. 390). In these cases, status as a person is granted through the authority of science as it is embodied in textbooks and international "consensus."

In addition to uses of scientific authority, several individuals use the language of biology to claim that embryos are humans. Some use the language of biological classification. Dr. Micheline Mathews-Roth of Harvard Medical School repeatedly describes embryos as the "youngest members of our species" (*Stem Cell Research, part 3,* 2000, p. 68), and Nigel Cameron from the Centre for Bioethics and Public Policy says, "My point is that the early human embryo is a member of the human species" (*Stem Cells, 2001,* 2001, p. 109). Species identity—classification of an organism as a human, although the basis for that classification is unspecified—becomes the basis for human identity and legal protection. A similar set of claims uses the language of growth and development. For Dr. Christopher Hook, "the human embryo is a person in an early phase of maturation through which every one of us has passed. She is not some other species. She is not merely tissue. Tissue cannot continue to develop into a full human being" (*Opportunities and Advancements,* 2001, p. 180). Russell Saltzman draws out the various stages of human development: "We all once sprang from an act of union between egg and sperm. We all once were human embryos. We all once were fetuses quickening in our mother's womb. We are all, each, human life" (*Stem Cell Research, part 3,* 2000, p. 97). For Hook and Saltzman, identity between embryos and developed humans is predicated on the fact that each has gone, or will go, through the same stages of development. Father Kevin Fitzgerald also develops a continuum of human development, but he ties it to an increase in the number of cells in the body: "As a human being continues to develop as a fetus, infant, child and adult, the number of cells in the body increases" (*Stem Cell Research,* 2001, p. 76). For Fitzgerald, the difference between the embryo and the adult is a difference of degree—the number of extant cells—and not a difference of kind. Biological classification and human development provide the basis for identifying embryos as human beings, and that identification then becomes the basis for extending legal protections and rights to them.

Finally, speakers supplement these continua with repetition and emotional language when describing how ES cells are isolated. The prepared testimony of the Center for Bioethics and Human Dignity repeatedly uses the terms "destruction" and "death" to describe the derivation of ES cells (*Opportunities and Advancements,* 2001, pp. 388–394). While the valence of destruction is still somewhat ambiguous, "death" implies the humanity of the embryo used to derive ES cells, and the use of "death" alongside the word "destruction" gives the latter term a negative valence. Both Dr. Christopher Hook and Eric Salley, who testify before the House Committee on Government Reform's subcommittee on criminal justice, drug policy, and human resources, use the phrase "living human embryos" multiple times, and the prepared testimonies of John and Lucinda Borden and Marlene Strege refer to the derivation of ES cells as "slaughter" and "genocide" (*Opportunities and Advancements,* 2001). While these emotional images do not have explicit biological connotations, the most commonly used image for deriving ES cells—harvesting—provides the grounds for biological readings. As noted earlier, "harvesting" implies agriculture and a view of embryonic life as a product. Richard Doerflinger states, "Harvesting the embryonic stem cells is not done after the embryo is killed; it is precisely what kills the embryo" (*Stem Cell Research,* 1999, p. 137n12). According to Dr. Frank Young, a former director of the Food and Drug Administration (FDA), "killing embryos by disintegration to harvest stem cells is illegal, immoral and unnecessary" (*Stem Cell Research, part 2,* 1999, p. 5). Joann Davidson, director of Snowflakes Embryo Adoption Program, opposes the "destruction of human embryos for any purpose, including the lethal 'harvesting' and medical experimentation upon the stem cells that compose each living human embryo" (*Opportunities and Advancements,* 2001, p. 82). The implication of agriculture and a view of embryonic life as a product is explicitly drawn out by Sen. Sam Brownback in a discussion of ES cells and therapeutic cloning: "Therapeutic cloning is where you take the young embryo . . . and then harvest—and I use that term again because we are almost talking in livestock terms here—harvest the stem cells" (*Stem Cells, 2001,* 2001, p. 20). Finally, the most thorough deployment of the harvesting metaphor comes from Mary Jane Owen of the National Catholic Office for Persons with

Disabilities (*Stem Cell Research, part 3,* 2000, pp. 27–29). She begins by urging the senators, "Do not, in the name of progress for disabled people, certify or justify the destructive harvesting of human embryos for stem cell research" (p. 26). From there, she argues that many Americans believe "human embryos and fetuses should not be harvested lest they come to be seen as products for sale" (p. 26) and that "most of us consider the idea of harvesting fellow human beings for the advantage of the few as abhorrent" (p. 26). Finally, she pleads, "We need you, members of the United States Senate, to call for a nationwide calming of the frenzied research efforts based upon destroying future citizens, rather than endorsing this national anxiety" (p. 28). Owen draws out the series of human forms throughout her testimony: She moves from concern about embryos, to "fetuses and embryos." Those fetuses are "fellow human beings," and finally "future citizens." This series ties the fate of the embryo to legal protections of persons and "citizens," and it is supported by the repetition of emotional language. She uses the figure of "harvesting" human life 11 times to describe the treatment of embryos or the unborn. The repetition of harvesting helps tie together the scattered elements of the series as a whole. It condemns the treatment of human life as an agricultural product that can be harvested and used by us for our own ends. The repetition of words like "harvest" with different stages of human development—fetuses, embryos, children, adult, "citizens," etc.—makes the actions done to any of these beings equivalent: Harvesting embryos, therefore, is the same as harvesting children or adults. The harvesting metaphor's organic and agricultural implications are consonant with an emphasis on biology, and the use of this metaphor, alongside the use of scientific language and references to scientific authority, helps to intensify the biorhetoric used by opponents of ES cell research.

Conclusion

Opponents of ES cell research find it difficult to challenge the "promise" of stem cell research directly. They turn to the abortion debate as their resource for inventing arguments for the ES cell debate. Their use of those resources and the journalistic coverage of them highlights the interplay between Manichean and scientistic idioms of public argument.

Journalistic uses of abortion as scene highlight the challenge of translating concerns from one idiom to another. Journalists use the abortion issue to render the ES cell debate intelligible: It becomes the scene within which the stem cell drama plays out. Yet, a simple understanding of the scene fails to account for prominent pro-life politicians who support this research, so some journalists use a rhetorical *paradox,* in which the apparent contradiction of pro-life politicians supporting ES cell research reveals a scene of greater ethical complexity. Furthermore, such a scene defines the opponents' objections to ES cell research as primarily religious. On the one hand, this is not a problematic explanation and is accurate for many of the people who speak out against the research, but it makes the debate one of religious objections to scientific progress. It also means that opponents would experience difficulty trying to make real definitions of embryos or ES cells that establish the terms of the debate in their favor.

In political discourse, opponents of ES cell discourse distance themselves from the abortion debate and turn to a combination of a scientistic idiom and biorhetoric. The scientistic idiom's real definitions create the *is*—the statement of fact—from which biorhetoric derives its *ought*—the moral position opposing ES cell research because of the harm done to embryos. This moral argument is made here, as in the journalistic discourse, through the use of the public fetus, a rhetorical figure from the abortion debate that collapses all developing human life into the figure of the "unborn baby" who is treated as the equivalent of born, rights-bearing individuals. Yet, the political discourse of the opposition combines and intensifies the scientistic idiom and biorhetoric: Opponents turn to the language of biology and genetics to support their case, instead of relying on moral and religious backing for their claims.

This turn to the language of science represents an intensification of the biorhetoric in this debate—the tendency to dress one's ethical claims in scientific fact. The presumption that science has a "chaste," value-free rhetoric is problematic in its own right, and the use of biorhetorical strategies predicated on an image of chaste scientific rhetoric is a problematic strategy for opponents of ES cell research. As we saw above, the use of science to support the opposition claim that ES cells *were* embryos did not succeed, and as we shall see in the next chapter, proponents also have a number of arguments that counter the use of the public fetus and that also intensify the biorhetoric of this debate while building on the proponents' scientific ethos.

4
Blastocysts, Spare Embryos, and Embryo Adoption
Redefining the Beginnings of Human Life

Opponents turn to the public fetus, a key rhetorical figure from the abortion debate, to help make their case against ES cell research. Because some scientific and cultural practices have destabilized the public fetus, the public fetus and the rights of actual humans must be explicitly extended to the 14-day-old blastocyst from which ES cells are derived in order for opponents to successfully argue against federal funding for ES cell research. This extension has highlighted the challenge of translating definition grounded in religious discourse into a scientistic idiom; and the resulting discourse combines a scientistic discourse, establishing the *fact* of an embryo's personhood, with a biorhetorical element, in which a *normative* stance was derived from the fact of personhood.

Yet, this need to extend the public fetus also highlights the argumentative space where *proponents* can attempt to circumvent or defuse the public fetus's power: The need for explicit extension means that disrupting the power of the public fetus is possible. Proponents use two arguments to disrupt the extension of the public fetus to ES cell debates. The first is a pragmatic argument about the existence of "spare embryos," embryos produced by in vitro fertilization (IVF) that are in excess of a couple's reproductive needs. The second involves redefining "embryo" so that it no longer refers to the blastocyst and earlier embryonic forms. In doing so, proponents follow the same path as opponents of research, producing a discourse that blurs the scientistic idiom with biorhetorical elements.

Spare Embryos and Embryo Adoption

The argument extending the status of person from the late-term fetus to the embryo develops out of a powerful cultural logic, but proponents of ES cell research have developed responses that attempt to circumvent or defuse its power. Here I discuss how proponents try to create an exception to this logic by raising the issue of "orphan" or "spare embryos." As noted in the previous chapter, the process of IVF creates embryos in excess of many couples' reproductive needs. This raises issues of whether the embryos are life or property and how to handle their use and, typically, their disposal. Proponents of ES cell research emphasize either that spare embryos remain frozen until they are destroyed or that the time spent frozen damages their capacity to develop. Opponents respond to these arguments with three different strategies: They reiterate the moral status of the embryo, argue that the number of "spare embryos" created can be manipulated by scientists, and argue that spare embryos can be adopted.

Pragmatic Arguments about Spare Embryos

During the first hearing on embryonic stem cell research, bioethicist Arthur Caplan summarizes the status of IVF and embryo overproduction. His presentation establishes the three components of the pragmatic argument about spare embryos: "This country now finds itself in a situation in which tens of thousands of orphan embryos sit in liquid nitrogen unwanted and highly unlikely to be used by anyone ever to try to make babies" (*Stem Cell Research,* 1999, p. 39). Caplan's testimony depicts these embryos as superfluous, and he argues that this condition removes them from the category of potential human beings. Next, Caplan argues against the claim that spare embryos, because they are *embryos,* still represent life:

> There are some who would still object that these frozen embryos are still potential persons. But that claim does not square with the facts. If no woman is willing to have the embryos placed inside her bodies [*sic*], if clinics are reluctant to use embryos that have been stored for long periods of time because their potential to become babies is diminished or if couples do not want anyone else using their embryos then their potential for becoming persons is zero. (p. 39)

Because these embryos are superfluous, they cannot be potential persons: Either they will never be implanted in a woman's uterus and allowed to develop, or they will lose their capacity to develop as a result of long-term storage. Caplan concludes, "Spare embryos would seem to be a legitimate and morally defensible source of human embryonic stem cells" (p. 39). Caplan presents the fullest version of this argument. He identifies the situation of IVF and the overproduction of embryos in the United States, defines those embryos as something other than human life (and thus lacking legal rights), and argues on the basis of that definition that using them in ES cell research is legitimate. This is an argument from definition: The second set of claims about embryos being something other than human represents the crux of the definition, and accepting those claims leads to the conclusions that Caplan makes. Other journalistic and political discourse uses some of the same claims Caplan deploys, but very few discuss all three with the same detail. Instead, they engage in argument *by* definition and present fragments of the argument.[1] This allows the key definitional move either to appear as a matter of fact claim or to become an enthymematic conclusion drawn by the audiences themselves.[2]

Factual claims about the state of IVF and the number of spare embryos that exist appear in both political and journalistic discourse. Dr. James Thomson, who first isolated ES cells, identifies the situation with spare embryos and how that situation forced a decision on IVF patients: "[The embryos] were beyond what the patients could use. The majority of these embryos had been frozen for a number of years, and they had to decide what to do with them. The option that they were considering was to discard them, so it was a choice between discarding the embryos and doing this research" (*Stem Cell Research,* 1998, p. 28). Thomson's implications in presenting this situation undermine a view of spare embryos as equivalent to living human beings. Embryos exist in excess of the patient's need. Because the embryos were not used, they were slated for destruction. Parents were then faced with two options: pointless destruction or donation for research.

Identifying the existence of spare embryos at IVF clinics is very common in the journalistic coverage of this issue. Often, the status of embryos in IVF is described with a word or brief phrase. News reports describe "discarded embryos" ("Christopher Reeve Asks," 2000) or "frozen embryos" ("Complication," 2001). The use of these terms is meant to describe their condition—that they are left over from IVF attempts—but with the exception of "frozen," these terms also imply certain value judgments. "Discarded" implies that the embryos have been thrown away and that they have no value within the framework of IVF. Other terms used include "excess," "spare," and "surplus," all of which also imply that the embryos described are beyond the needs of the individuals who produced them, thus diminishing the embryos' perceived value. Finally, "donated" implies that these spare embryos do have value—they have been given up for research—and also that they have been given by those with the proper authority. Thus, in enumerating the "facts" about spare embryos, the description contains an ethical valuation that favors the use of spare embryos in ES cell research. Rather than establishing that something is real and arguing for a certain policy, these descriptions contain a moral valuation justifying specific courses of action. It is not just that ES cell research uses embryos stored in IVF facilities. Embryos have a moral status in being stored at an IVF facility, and that status, variously described as a state of being "discarded," "surplus," or "spare," justifies their use.

Newspaper coverage presents this issue using brief phrases describing the source of ES cells. *The Milwaukee Journal Sentinel* notes that ES cells come from "leftover embryos donated from infertility clinics" (Marchione, 2000). *The San Francisco Chronicle* explains, "Ideally, embryos for stem cell experiments would be leftovers from in-vitro fertilization" (Abate, 2000). Television news blends the visual and discursive when making this claim by weaving together visual images from IVF clinics or images of microscopic embryos with verbal presentation of information about stem cells or IVF. One NBC news segment shows science correspondent Robert Bazell dressed in hospital scrubs and walking through an IVF clinic. He stops by a large liquid nitrogen tank that presumably contains embryos and says, "No one knows the exact number, but in clinics across the country, liquid nitrogen containers like these contain between 300,000 and a million frozen human embryos—far more than enough to satisfy the needs of medical research" ("Jones Institute Recruits," 2001). A CNN report shows a liquid nitrogen tank used to store frozen embryos while a voice-over from medical correspondent Elizabeth Cohen notes, "In IVF clinics—those are fertility clinics around the country—they sit frozen in tanks like these. There are about 100,000 [*the number 100,000 appears at the bottom of the screen*]—maybe even more—in the country. These are again embryos sitting in fertility labs. 100,000 is a lot" ("President Bush Makes," 2001). Finally, in reporting that the Bush administration would soon announce its policy, Katie Couric begins the news report with a description of spare embryos and IVF that is delivered over a montage of images from IVF clinics that begins and ends with pictures of fertilized eggs: "These are tiny fertilized eggs, human embryos, the potential for human life or potentially life-saving cures. Hundreds of thousands created every year for infertile couples. Each couple may fertilize dozens of eggs. Only some are used. The rest, usually discarded" ("Debate over Stem Cell Research," 2001).

In each case, the images used do three things. First, they show that spare embryos exist. Second, the presentation of the storage conditions for these embryos—the fact that they exist in liquid nitrogen and not the womb—implies a set of value judgments about spare embryos, ranging from recognition that *some people, somewhere* do not value embryos to the conclusion that these embryos *in fact* do not have any value. Third, micrographs—images of microscopic objects taken with a microscope and camera—of spare embryos also contribute to later arguments that these embryos are not like actual human beings.

Explicit redefinition of what counts as an "embryo" so that the concept of "spare embryos" no longer falls in that category does not appear in the political discourse, outside of Caplan's initial argument in 1998, and it appears very rarely in the journalistic coverage of the debate. One article refers to a decision by President Clinton's National Bioethics Advisory Commission that described deriving stem cells from spare embryos as "morally akin to removing organs for transplant from dead people who had consented" (Ackerman, 2001). A *New York Times* article explains how "large numbers of these futureless embryos are stored in freezers throughout the country" (Wade, 2001a). The most extensive use of explicit redefinition appears in *The Atlanta Journal-Constitution*:

> The harsh realities of infertility treatment also make it hard to view those embryos as fully human. Once fertilized, the vast majority of embryos that are returned to the womb never develop into a human baby. The rate is so low that doctors at RBA [Reproductive Biology Associates] return as many as four embryos at a time to the womb, in hopes that just one will implant and develop.
>
> Those embryos not immediately returned to the womb are frozen, in case the first treatment fails to produce a pregnancy. Unfortunately, the success rate with those embryos is even lower than with freshly fertilized eggs. (Bookman, 2001)

Each article highlights a condition or quality that renders problematic the definition of "spare embryos" as human life, whether that is an analogy to dead people from whom organs are harvested for transplant or the fact that examining the reality of fertility treatments reveals that spare embryos are "futureless"—that they will never become people.

Explicit argument from definition is rare, probably because explicitly proffering a definition about the status of embryonic life invites controversy. Explicit attempts to argue from definition would rapidly become arguments *about* definitions. Given the political sensitivity of ES cell research, politicians wish to avoid appearing cavalier about the moral concerns people have about the beginnings of human life, and given the journalistic standard of objectivity, controversial statements like these will usually be avoided by journalists who do not want to appear biased. Using an explicit argument about definition will be difficult and often avoided, but if the definition is stipulated in passing or presented as a fact of the situation—in other words, as argument *by* definition—then the claim can be made to appear less controversial. Thus, reporters refer to the facts of IVF practice and pronouncements by national commissions, and they deploy brief descriptive phrases instead of presenting the definition at the crux of this argument.

Defining the ethical course of action is the most common approach to arguments about spare embryos as an appropriate source for ES cells. Proponents argue that spare embryos will never be used to produce children and that they are almost always discarded. In a *USA Today* article from May 1999, the head of

President Clinton's National Bioethics Advisory Commission claims, "There is a consensus forming that it is permissible to conduct this type of research on embryos left over from [in vitro fertilization] procedures where they would have been discarded in any event" (Friend, 1999). A CBS news segment from July 2001 reports, "At least three antiabortion Senators and scores of Republicans have urged the President to approve funding where abortion is not involved. Those cells would come from excess embryos created by in vitro fertilization" ("President Bush Continues Vacation," 2001). A 2001 *Seattle Times* article says, "Surplus frozen embryos in storage at fertility clinics, which are no longer wanted by the couples who had created them, are the most widely accepted source of embryos by scientists" ("Here's What Debate," 2001). These news reports couch the claim that using spare embryos in research is ethical as an issue of "permissibility" and "acceptability."

Typically, individuals defining the ethical course of action contrast it with the image of individuals discarding embryos. Specifically, they contrast discarding embryos with possible medical uses of the embryos' stem cells, creating the impression that the option is to either discard embryos and fail to help people with illnesses, or donate the embryos for vital medical research. Christopher Reeve asks, "Is it more ethical for a woman to donate unused embryos that will never become human beings, or to let them be tossed away as so much garbage when they could help save thousands of lives?" (*Stem Cell Research, part 3,* 2000, p. 36).[3] Dr. Richard Hynes says, "I submit that if the issue is morality, using embryonic stem cells for life-saving research is greatly preferable to discarding them" (*Stem Cell Research, part 3,* 2000, p. 85). Senator Orrin Hatch asks, "Why shouldn't these embryos slated for destruction be used for the good of mankind?" (*Opportunities and Advancements,* 2001, p. 14).[4] The image of dumping embryos into the trash encapsulates the argument for using spare embryos in ES cell research. Spare embryos are superfluous embryos. They will not become a human life. IVF clinics dispose of most, if not all, spare embryos. Therefore, according to the argument, using them in ES cell research is morally justifiable.

Proponents also use the routine discarding of spare embryos to attack pro-life opponents of ES cell research by claiming those opponents hold an incoherent position. During an exchange about the moral status of IVF, Senator Tom Harkin remarks, "Well, again I think, I can understand if you were opposed to in vitro fertilization, then I can see it [opposition to the use of spare embryos in research], but if you are for it, then you have got to say, okay, what do you do with these leftover?" (*Stem Cell Research, part 3,* 2000, p. 106). Proponents ask this question in order to highlight what they see as a contradiction in the position of many opponents of ES cell research. If opponents support IVF, the argument goes, they support the creation of spare embryos that are not accorded the respect opponents attach to embryonic life. The question becomes more pointed, and the appearance of contradiction greater, if the individual does not raise objections to the destruction of spare embryos from IVF clinics while still opposing ES cell research.

Television news, in addition to using footage from congressional testimonies, often uses footage in which ill or physically disabled individuals present this argument. Christopher Reeve makes this argument often. During an interview with NBC's Brian Williams, Reeve says, "We don't want to create embryos just for research. We want to rescue these cells from the garbage" ("George Bush Visits," 2001). In an interview with CBS in the days before President Bush announces his decision, Reeve argues, "90% or more [of individuals who have used IVF] decide that they simply are going to let these embryos be thrown away. If you believe that life begins at the moment of fertilization, and the state licenses these institutions to do that, technically speaking, you've got state-sanctioned murder. One in 6 couples conceive [*sic*] that way. You can be pro-life and pro-stem cells" ("Whether Stem Cell Research," 2001). The use of individuals like Reeve to present this argument intensifies the dilemma between choosing to save spare embryos and choosing to help the sick. Reeve acts as a visual reminder of the promise of medical applications from ES cell research while he presents the verbal argument that spare embryos will be destroyed, whether they are used for ES cell research or not. Verbally, he presents the argument that using spare embryos will not create an ethical harm, while he visually reminds audiences of the ethical benefits that can come from this research.

In contrast to television news, newspapers usually present this argument by quoting scientists. The most frequently used spokesperson for this argument is Dr. James Thomson, the scientist who first isolated human ES cells. A 1999 article from the Minneapolis *Star Tribune* quotes Dr. Thomson: "'Couples undergoing treatment for infertility sometimes create more embryos than they can use' he said. 'Typically they are discarded. In my mind, using such embryos that would otherwise be discarded was not only acceptable, but throwing them out when you could do something useful with them would be unacceptable'" (Schmickle, 1999a). An April 2000 article in *The Milwaukee Journal Sentinel* reports Thomson's attitude toward using spare embryos: "As he sees it, Thomson said, 'I'm not killing an embryo for research. I'm getting something useful out of something that's being thrown away'" (Ward, 2000). Later that year, *The Omaha World Herald* interviews Thomson, who again makes this case: "'Why would you throw them out?' he said. 'It's an ethically bad choice'" (Olson, 2000e). Newspaper coverage focuses on the ES cell researcher who rehearses a justification for undertaking controversial research in the first place, which then becomes the justification for continuing the research and providing expanded financial support for it.

Opposition Arguments about Spare Embryos

Opponents use one of three responses to the pragmatic argument about spare embryos. First, opponents argue that the distinction between "necessary" and "spare" embryos is meaningless and imply that IVF clinics will alter their methods in order to produce embryos to meet the needs of researchers. During the first hearing on stem cell research, Richard Doerflinger claimed, "We found a number of statements from people who run the IVF clinics who were willing to say that the distinction was meaningless. Basically, if you allow the research on spare embryos, then when they do the IVF work, the in vitro fertilization work, they will just make more of them up front and make sure that they will have spares left after the fact" (*Stem Cell Research,* 1999, p. 70). Dr. Usala makes a similar point in a 2000 hearing: "Science is an all-consuming fire. What will happen is, maybe a few more embryos will be fertilized so that we could give the embryos to justifiably sound science for development. . . . It will lead to that, if we state as the precedent that the use of embryos in this way is in and of itself okay" (*Stem Cell Research, part 3,* 2000, p. 103). The Minneapolis *Star Tribune* reports opponents' claims that the argument for using spare embryos in research "only makes sense in the context of a technology that already has gone too far by allowing embryos to be created and then discarded" (Schmickle, 2000a). *The Milwaukee Journal Sentinel* reports the concerns of the local Right to Life organization that "too many embryos are being created for fertility purposes, and that restrictions need to be placed on that because ultimately many of those embryos are being destroyed" (Schubert & Fauber, 2000a). In journalistic and political arenas, opponents try to undermine views of some embryos as "spare" or extraneous. In the congressional discourse, both Doerflinger and Usala create a slippery slope toward a dark future: If ES cell research goes forward, the demand for embryos will increase; the people who run IVF clinics are weak or evil, and they will create more embryos to meet demand. Embryos become spare because of the voracious and unethical needs of scientific research. For the opponents quoted in the journalistic discourse, the present time and present activity of IVF clinics is problematic: Life is created in IVF clinics only to be destroyed needlessly.

A second argument compares spare embryos and prisoners on death row. For example, Ron Heagy, president and founder of the Life Is an Attitude Foundation, argues, "The frozen embryos are potential human life right now. If you thaw them out and let them die, then they are dead, correct, and prisoners, and like—what we are discussing, yes, they have a voice right now, but once they are executed they are dead, so why can we not take their parts. It is the same thought process in my mind" (*Stem Cell Research, part 3,* 2000, p. 108). Father Kevin Fitzgerald also uses this argument:

> Who among us has the right to decide that another human life is a 'spare' life, especially when that human life does not have the chance to contest the decision? We do not consider it appropriate to take organs from dying patients or prisoners on "death row" before they have died in order to increase someone else's chances for healing or cure. Neither, then, should we consider any embryos "spare" so that we may destroy them for their stem cells. (*Stem Cell Research,* 2001, p. 77)

Comparisons of actual people with potential people develop out of a rhetorical strategy that extends personhood to all stages of developing life, making them the equivalent of people who have been born. This comparison is based, in part, on biology: For example, Fitzgerald's comparison of prisoners and embryos follows his claim that the difference between embryos and adults is the number of cells present in both (see chapter 3).

Finally, some opponents of ES research offer the practice of "embryo adoption" as a counterargument to the idea of spare embryos. This alternative is discussed at length during a hearing by the House Government Reform Committee's subcommittee on criminal justice, drug reform, and human resources. In embryo adoption, couples acquire legal ownership or custody of spare embryos and attempt to have them thawed and implanted. Those who discuss embryo adoption use many of the same strategies that appear when speakers establish the personhood of the embryo. Repetition is used, and an emphasis on embryos as children predominates. For example, Joann Davidson, director of Snowflakes Embryo Adoption Program, says, "Snowflakes like human embryos are frozen, unique and cannot be recreated" (*Opportunities and Advancements,* 2001, p. 74). She then repeats the phrase "frozen live humans" three times in her testimony. The children who are the result of embryo adoption were brought to this hearing and used as visual condensation symbols for the argument. While describing her daughter Hannah, Marlene Strege states, "No mere 'dot,' she contained within her the entire blueprint for human life, including all her human organs and tissues" (*Opportunities and Advancements,* 2001, p. 43). John and Lucinda Borden say, "Mark and Luke are living rebuttal to the claim that embryos are not people" (*Opportunities and Advancements,* 2001, p. 50).

Claims about embryo adoption also appear in a handful of journalistic sources. *USA Today* quotes Rep. Tom DeLay (R-TX): "'Nothing is more heart-wrenching than to see those little 'snowflakes' brought into a hearing room'" (Kiely &

Hall, 2001). Another *USA Today* article quotes Rep. Chris Smith (R–NJ), who describes the liquid nitrogen tanks at IVF clinics as a "frozen orphanage" (Keen & Welch, 2001). The three television news stories addressing embryo adoption all present the story of the Borden family and the embryos that became their twin sons, Mark and Luke. An ABC report from July 9, 2001, presents images of the Borden family during their everyday routine. The news segment begins with close-ups of the Borden twins, while correspondent Terry Moran announces in a voice-over, "These are two of the human faces of the stem cell debate— Mark and Luke Borden, nine-month-old twins, who were adopted when they were frozen embryos." Later, the segment shows Lucinda Borden being interviewed at home: "Adoption is respect of that life. And putting these children up for adoption is a much better way to respect that life than donating them for research and killing them off" ("Debate in the White House," 2001). The statement creates a jarring contrast between respecting the lives of unborn children versus "killing them off," which is made more intense by the contrast between the harsh description of ES cell research and the familial settings presented visually. A similar remark is made by father John Borden at a congressional hearing. While holding his two sons, he asks, "Which one of my children would you kill? Which one would you choose to take? Would you want to take Luke, the giggler, who we call 'Turbo,' or do you want to take the big guy, 'Tank'? Which one would you take?" ("Stem Cell Research Debate," 2001; see also "Stem Cell Research," 2001).

Arguments about embryo adoption do three things. First, the "snowflake" image emphasizes the fragility and uniqueness of spare embryos. Second, the language of "killing" aims to evoke an emotional reaction to the use of spare embryos in research. Third, these claims derive their power from the series logic noted earlier: If the children present today who came from adopted embryos are people, their point of origin—spare embryos—must be people.

Biorhetoric and the Scientistic Idiom in Spare Embryo Arguments

Discussion of "spare embryos" aims to carve out an exception to the definition of embryos as people. During the normal course of operations in an IVF clinic, these spare embryos will *never become* actual human beings. While part of the argument is based on how IVF is practiced, another part of it—that frozen embryos lose their capacity to develop over time—grounds the status of embryos in a biological condition, the impossibility of development. The opposition response to the spare embryo argument is also open to biological interpretation. The comparison of prisoners and embryos depends on creating a rhetorical series, which, as noted earlier, is often grounded in biology. In saying that the embryo that became her daughter is a person, Marlene Strege bases her claim on the embryo's DNA—the blueprint for human life. In most cases, these arguments are presented as facts, and the presentation of these facts incorporates a biorhetorical element, which is intensified by the use of repetition and emotional language.

Countering the Personhood of the Embryo

Some proponents of embryonic stem cell research, like Senator Arlen Specter (R-PA), respond to the argument for embryo adoption on pragmatic grounds that the number of embryos "saved" by adoption cannot match the number of embryos destroyed in the everyday practice of IVF clinics (*Stem Cell Research,* 2001, p. 123). Yet, this response leaves unanswered concerns about the personhood of the embryo. Proponents of ES cell research therefore also use a set of rhetorical strategies that circulate out from scientists and congressional testimony and that create a new class of embryo, which lacks status as a person.

The first strategy involves distinguishing between two categories—embryos that will develop and embryos that will not develop. Bioethicist Arthur Caplan notes, "Most human embryos at the point of conception will not become human beings even under the best of all possible developmental circumstances. . . . While it is true as a matter of historical fact that all human life has begun with conception it is not true that all conception is capable of becoming human life" (*Stem Cell Research,* 1999, p. 38). Senator Hatch makes a similar distinction: "I believe that a human's life begins in the womb, not a petri dish or refrigerator" (*Opportunities and Advancements,* 2001, p. 14). An article in *The Chicago Sun-Times* notes, "Scientists object to automatically equating an embryo with an aborted fetus" ("Embryo Research Debated," 1998). *The Milwaukee Journal Sentinel* quotes Dr. Caplan: "At the point of implantation, an embryo's 'moral status changes,' Caplan said. 'The crucial moment is implantation, not conception,' because many embryos are flawed and not viable, he said" (Marchione, 1998). An article in *USA Today* reports on scientific observations of embryos and the conclusions scientists draw: "Scientists say blastocysts often do not survive past the first 2 weeks of development. Because of that fact, some scientists and religious groups do not regard blastocysts with the same status as embryos that are in the womb and have begun developing anatomical features" (Friend, 2001f).

As Caplan notes in his testimony and in his newspaper interview, human life begins at conception, but not all conceptions are human life. Many early-stage embryos do not implant into the uterus and never become life. Some groups say these pre-implantation embryos do not have the same status as life at later developmental stages, and if an embryo remains, as Hatch says, in the "refrigerator," then it will never have the opportunity to develop. These arguments attempt to break apart the continuum of personhood created by opponents and redefine those parts as two unique categories. The creation of these two categories—embryos that will become life and embryos that will not—allows rhetors to argue that research with human embryos in the second category is permissible.

A second strategy emphasizes the visual differences between fully developed humans and embryos. Some of these arguments focus on the size of the embryo in order to emphasize its lack of similarity to human beings. Dr. Mary Hendrix claims, "This very early embryo (called the blastocyst) is so small that it can fit on the tip of a sewing needle" (*Stem Cells, 2001,* 2001, p. 56). Often discussion of size is connected to a lack of other obviously human features. In her September 2000 testimony, Mary Tyler Moore, actress and chairwoman of the Juvenile Diabetes Foundation, states, "The embryos that are being discussed, according to science, bears [*sic*] as much resemblance to a human being as a goldfish" (*Stem Cell Research, part 3,* 2000, p. 120). Later, in the hearing, Senator Harkin follows up on her comment: "I think a lot of people get confused, thinking an embryo is something, almost like a fetus or something like that, a fully developed fetus. We are talking about something less than the size of a pencil dot" (p. 121). Finally, Dr. Bert Vogelstein makes a similar claim about embryos: "They have none of the characteristics of human beings. It's essential to distinguish a human being from human cells" (*Cloning,* 2001, p. 34).

Journalists often report on the lack of visual similarity without making explicit judgment. CBS's medical correspondent Elizabeth Kaledin describes embryos as "the tiny bundles of cells, no bigger than a pencil point" ("Influential Senator Bill Frist," 2001). *USA Today* describes a blastocyst as "a ball of cells the size of a pinhead" (Kiely & Hall, 2001). The *Star Tribune* notes that a blastocyst "consists of a sphere of cells with an outer layer, a fluid-filled cavity and an inner cell mass" (Schmickle, 1999a), and *The Atlanta Journal-Constitution* states, "The political, ethical and religious furor created by the question of allowing federal funding of embryonic stem cell research comes down to some tiny little pinkish-yellow bumps in a Petri dish" (Guthrie, 2001). Rarely do journalists move beyond description of early-stage embryos to the conclusions drawn by proponents. *The Houston Chronicle* does quote a local expert who observes, "It really looks nothing like a human" (Dooley, 2001), while the authors of a 2000 *Milwaukee Journal Sentinel* article claim in their own voice, "They [blastocysts] had not yet begun to make the cells that distinguish a human being" (Schubert & Fauber, 2000b; also see Wade, 2000b).

Arguments about the size and characteristics of the embryo emphasize the dissimilarity between embryos and full-grown humans and late-term fetuses.

Even the relatively neutral journalistic descriptions highlight the differences between the two. Embryos have no human organs or other "characteristics," and they are so small they cannot be seen with the naked eye. Whether an explicit conclusion about the personhood of an embryo is drawn or not, the emphasis on these differences distances the embryo from fully developed humans. It also represents an intensification of the biorhetorical components of the debate: Claims about physical characteristics are organized and presented in a way to insinuate an ethical and social message about the personhood of developing life.

Third, proponents argue that recent scientific developments—especially somatic cell nuclear transfer (SCNT), the basis for cloning—have made previous conceptions of the embryo and the beginnings of human life moot. This strategy appears only in congressional testimony and not news reports, possibly because it requires presenting a high degree of technical information, from which journalists might shy away, and because it raises issues around other controversial scientific discoveries like cloning. This strategy claims that embryos are only potential life, and that since SCNT makes it possible for things like hair and skin to become potential human beings, the category "potential human life" has distinctly less value. In the first hearing on embryonic stem cell research, Caplan claims, "Some of the bright lines that we think we can go to are not so bright when the DNA of any cell can be converted ultimately, potentially, to a human being by transfer and technology that allows for nuclear cell cloning. We can no longer say that we understand exactly when life begins, how to respect life, depending on certain properties that might inhere in particular cells or tissues" (*Stem Cell Research,* 1999, pp. 36–37). Dr. Ron Green from Dartmouth College's Ethics Institute notes, "In an era of cloning technology, every single cell in our body has the potential to be equated with these clusters of cells [i.e., embryos]" (*Cloning,* 2001, p. 33). Dr. Bert Vogelstein uses an extended example to make the point:

I could take a—skin cells from a little biopsy or cheek cells, or I could even take a hair. Now, is that hair a clone of me? It's not such a trivial question, because each cell in the hair is genetically identical to me, to every other cell in my body, and moreover, the cells in that hair have the potential to be me. It used to be, just a few years ago, thought that there was a strict line between the potential to form human life and human life, and that potential was only in embryos. But we now know that every living cell in an animal's body could at least potentially be used to create human life. And it's very important to discriminate the potential for human life from real human life. (*Cloning,* 2001, p. 24)

All three men emphasize that cloning technologies make it possible for any cell to become human life. Yet those cells would not be treated as people. We do not allow hairs, to use Vogelstein's example, to have any of the rights or privileges we attach to people or citizens. By foregrounding the potential of *any* cell to become the beginnings of human life, this argument lowers the value of potential life because of the sundry cell types that occupy that category.

The fourth strategy is also based in biology, but uses the findings of embryology to argue for a biologically based distinction between people and the potential life of blastocysts and other embryonic forms. In response to calls for a bright line separating ethical and unethical research on embryos, proponents of ES cell research suggest using the primitive streak, the proto-spinal cord that appears on the 15th day after conception, when the embryo implants in the uterine wall. Dr. Michael West argues,

> The bright line [that], I would argue, would be a wise one for us to draw is primitive streak. At about the time of implantation, this pre-implantation embryo begins the first steps toward becoming a human being, or indeed it may form two human beings, identical twins. Primitive streak, I think, is an effective line to draw and say that is the beginning of a human being. And prior to primitive streak we should use some other terminology, a pre-implantation embryo or some other such terminology, because this is not an individualized human being. (*Cloning,* 2001, p. 15)

West argues that the primitive streak separates an embryo, which West identifies as a person, from a pre-implantation embryo, which is a group of cells with human DNA that is not a human person. West reiterates this point later in the same hearing, but this time, he argues that the division is natural and not manmade:

> And our point is, there is such a convenient line, a bright line that we could draw, which is drawn for us by nature itself. It's called primitive streak. So once this cluster of cells attaches and finds a home in a woman's uterus, to begin a pregnancy, nature begins by drawing a line on those cells. It's called primitive streak, it's the first—it's sort of the spade in the ground, you know, the ceremonial spade to start the construction of the building. It's the first step towards the production, the beginnings of a human life. A human life, as opposed to what was cellular life. (*Cloning,* 2001, p. 33)

In addition to repeating the phrase "primitive streak" multiple times, West transforms a social determination of when life begins or should be accorded legal rights and protection into a biological fact: The primitive streak, which appears

14 days after conception, marks the beginning of human life. This is an intensification of the biorhetoric and the scientistic idiom proponents are using, and it leads to scientism: Nature, not people, draws the dividing line between human life and human cells, and science divines the actions of nature and passes them on to the public.

Journalists couch discussion of the primitive streak and what embryonic forms count as human life in terms of development. *The Star Tribune* quotes a local expert in philosophy: "As the human conceptive—the embryo and fetus—develops, it gradually acquires greater moral significance" (Schmickle, 1999a). *USA Today* claims that many proponents of ES cell research "argue that life begins at a later stage of development" (Friend, 2001e). An article in *The Boston Globe* describes the development of the primitive streak as the moment when an embryo acquires a soul:

> There are also stem cell researchers who believe ensoulment occurs quite early, but later than the blastocyst stage. They point out that a blastocyst still has potential to become twins. How, then, can it have a soul? They believe as soon as the stem cells start on their missions and faint signs of a person appear, then ensoulment occurs. In this camp, many believe three weeks into a pregnancy, when the spine emerges, is the magic threshold. (Mishra, 2001c)

The claims from *The Star Tribune* and *USA Today* recapitulate the biorhetoric from congressional testimony: "Moral significance" and "life" become tied to biological development. The treatment of this argument in *The Boston Globe* represents a complicated negotiation of religious and scientific discourses. The key issue in this presentation of the debate is the issue of the soul: If embryos have souls, then ES cell research involves killing life. Yet, the earliest stages of embryonic life can still become twins, so the belief that the blastocyst and other early embryonic forms have "souls" becomes problematic. The loss of this capacity to twin becomes a "magic" threshold after which the soul appears. While still tying moral categories to a biological condition, this treatment of the debate blurs morality and biology together in the language of souls and magic, rendering a strictly biorhetorical or scientistic reading of the argument problematic.

Each of these arguments about the moral status of the earliest stages of life does two things. First, these strategies work to disrupt the rhetorical series used by opponents of this research to encourage identification with the embryo. They create a division between embryos and humans, a category that includes late-term fetuses. The first three arguments claim that embryos cannot be in the same category with other later forms of humanity because of gross physical differences. Arguments about cloning and the primitive streak work to cement that division by providing a "deeper" biological understanding of early human forms like the embryo and the blastocyst. These strategies reshape understandings of potential human life: That life used to be unique and precious, but the fact that potential exists in skin cells as well as embryos devalues potential and gives preference and value to actual human lives, those who have been born or who are almost ready to be born (that is, late-term fetuses).

Second, these strategies blend a scientistic idiom and biorhetoric. Proponents mesh statements about science and the physical world into social and ethical arguments so that "scientific" claims about the attributes of embryos equate to a moral position that distinguishes two different classes of embryos. While most journalistic presentations of these arguments do not explicitly endorse the conclusions proponents make, they ultimately contribute to the arguments' strength by keeping them in circulation. Additionally, proponents intensify the biorhetoric in these arguments into a type of scientism when they claim with the primitive streak that nature itself provides the determination of personhood, which scientists then discover.

From Abortion to Biorhetoric to Scientism

Proponents attempt to redefine what "embryo" means and the moral import it has for ES cell research. These redefinitions range from arguments about "spare embryos" to claims that a distinct class of embryos exists that do not deserve the same rights as people and late-term fetuses. These arguments—and the use of the public fetus discussed in the previous chapter—combine a scientistic idiom with biorhetoric: Rhetors in the debate define some quality of embryos or spare embryos as "real" and then derive an ethical precept from that fact. The proponents' arguments about spare embryos also *intensify* this process and transform it into a form of scientism.

As Lyne (1990) notes, people often connect discourses about what "is" to discourses about what "ought to be": Science, especially biology, has been used to frame our views of how we should act. This has been an operating principle of the public fetus: The "fact" of visual similarity between the fetus and us becomes the naturalistic framework for moral arguments against abortion. When it appears in congressional debates about ES cell research, the scientific component of the public fetus becomes intensified in ways that make it a scientism, a privileging of technical-scientific ways of knowing. In the ES cell debate, "ought" becomes replaced by "is." Statements about "natural," "objective," or "scientific" observations of fetuses and embryos become the primary trope in the debate.

Proponents also turn to scientism in arguments about the primitive streak. By describing the proto-spinal cord as *nature's* way of determining who is a person, scientists supporting ES cell research reduce a social and ethical argument about the beginnings of human life into a purely biological determination. This is not to say that using the primitive streak as a means of determining what kind of embryos can be used for experimentation is bad. Rather its mode of presentation distorts ethical decision making into a quasi-scientific determination. While scientism helps proponents make their case about ES cells, it ultimately disenfranchises all nonscientists, including nonscientific proponents of ES cell research, by making scientific expertise the necessary prerequisite for speaking on this issue. This differs from the scientistic idiom in that any individual who can couch their concerns in scientific language can use the idiom to create real definitions that shape the grounds for further debate. Scientism raises the bar for public discussion of science-based controversies, and thus becomes an issue of concern for individuals on both sides of this debate.

As this chapter and the previous one have shown, arguments about the embryo bolster scientism and treat ethical judgments as natural fact. Amplifying the scientistic idiom with biorhetorical appeals is problematic. Because more scientists support ES cell research, the use of biorhetoric and the scientistic idiom complicates attempts by some opponents to use language borrowed from biology to define ES cells as embryos and embryos as rights-bearing human beings. While *any* individual in principle has the capacity to use a scientistic idiom, supplementing it with biorhetorical appeals collapses value judgments into statements of fact and leaves open the possibility that rhetors affiliated with science will outmaneuver other rhetors and dominate public argument. If public argument collapses the process of establishing the facts of the matter and the process of determining the values that should be considered in a debate into one, unified mode of argument, then the possibilities for rich, multifaceted public debate on science-based controversies are foreclosed.

Finally, even if opponents of ES cell research could avoid some of these concerns about biorhetoric and the scientistic idiom, they face a daunting challenge in trying to establish a real definition of embryos as rights-bearing individuals. The objection that potential lives are destroyed by ES cell research does not persuade a large portion of the American public: When it comes to choosing between potential lives and actual lives, most Americans will choose to help those currently living. Therefore, opponents must supply additional lines of argument identifying a source of stem cells that is equally capable of producing medical applications. They turn, then, to arguments about adult stem cells and stem cell potency.

5
Power, Potency, and Plasticity
Hierarchies of Stem Cells and Their Inherent Ambiguities

One issue common to both the scientific and political debate about stem cell research is the issue of stem cell "potency"—the capacity of various stem cells to differentiate into the 210 tissues that constitute the human body. Over the course of the debate, rhetors increasingly focus on stem cell potency, the power to differentiate, as the key to attaining the three applications stem cell research promises. ES cells will supposedly fulfill all three applications, but it is possible that adult stem cells can be used to screen new drugs or as the source for medical applications. The debate over which cell type is "better" focuses on the degree of power or "potency" each group of cells supposedly has, and opponents continually emphasize the power of adult stem cells to supplement their arguments for banning ES cell research. If adult stem cells have equivalent power to ES cells, they argue, then morally troubling ES cell research is unnecessary.

Rhetors turn to several related terms to describe the degree of differentiation possible for each stem cell type. These range from totipotency, the capacity to produce all cell types, to pluripotency, and then multipotency before the range is restricted to the ability to produce only more of the same type of fully differentiated cell. This ranking of potency terms is one part of an argument from hierarchy in science. The potency terms provide the hierarchy used for organizing cell types, and rhetors use this hierarchy to generate claims about the value of different types of stem cells. Yet, the creation of hierarchy involves more than the creation of explicit ranks: Hierarchies also contain ambiguities and uncertainties that allow rhetors to blur the distinctions between a hierarchy's various levels.

Potency is the basis for the hierarchy of cell types. In the use of these potency hierarchies, we begin to see the overlap and interplay of science and the scientistic idiom, as well as support for Beck's (1992, p. 167) observation that public debate depends on scientific *language* but is divorced from specific scientific *findings*. Scientific and public rhetoric on the issues of potency uses the same set of terms and concepts to explain potency and define either ES cells as more potent than adult stem cells or adult stem cells as equivalent to ES cells in their potency. This overlap occurs in part because the scientific terms are not explicitly tied to specific experimental contexts and because the scientific terms draw their power from commonplace understandings of the word "potency" and the prefixes used to modify it. This allows for a relatively simple transition of terms between the public and scientific discourse.

Scientists develop rhetorical categories to distinguish the power various cells have and how that power can be used to attain the applications people desire. The hierarchy becomes the basis for scientific claims about which types of cells will provide the most efficacious path to applications. In public discourse found in congressional hearings and journalistic discourse, the hierarchy generates four types of claims. First, some discourse employs the hierarchy to emphasize the importance and power of ES cells. Second, some testimony deploys the ambiguities in the hierarchy to attack ES cell research and valorize adult stem cells. Third, some political rhetors use the interplay of opponents' attacks and the hierarchy to elaborate on the power of ES cells and reaffirm their greater place in stem cell hierarchies. And, finally, some rhetors create a series of ambivalent positions on stem cell research that emphasizes the uncertainty about the qualitative differences between adult stem and ES cells.

Hierarchy, Repetition, and Ambiguity: Creating Grounds for Argument

According to Perelman and Olbrechts-Tyteca (1969), the power of hierarchies lies in their capacity to act as a resource for, as well as the subject of, debate: "Hierarchies, like values, belong to the agreements which serve as premises to discourses. But hierarchies can also be the subject of argumentation; there can be discussion as to whether a hierarchy is well founded and where some one of its terms belongs" (p. 337). Jeanne Fahnestock (1999) notes that classical rhetoricians identified a variety of hierarchies used in argument. The most common form in both scientific and non-scientific argument is the *incrementum,* which embodies a principle of ordering or gradation. According to Fahnestock, rhetors can use the *incrementum* in a variety of ways. In two of the most common uses, a rhetor can create a series in order to organize a set of concepts, and "an arguer can also use an established series or hierarchy as a model for forming another" (Fahnestock, 1999, p. 97).

Using a preexisting series to organize another set of terms along the same lines is discussed in *The New Rhetoric* (Perelman & Olbrechts-Tyteca, 1969). Arguments from hierarchy, called double hierarchies by Perelman and Olbrechts-Tyteca, use an established or familiar hierarchy to form a second hierarchy and bring order to a new realm of objects: "The double hierarchy makes it possible to base a contested hierarchy on an accepted hierarchy" (p. 342). Arguments from hierarchy produce claims about order or rank among a group of objects or categories; a hierarchy helps rhetors define an object by comparing it to other objects. These hierarchies can be strengthened through repetition of key elements. That repetition creates a consistency in terminology that implies a consistency in the objects and categories discussed (Fahnestock, 1999; Perelman & Olbrechts-Tyteca, 1969). Repetitions also "provide visual chains across a text" (Fahnestock, 1999, p. 157). By repeating words, or the roots of words, throughout a text, an arguer creates the sense of unity among the (potentially) disparate objects being discussed together. That unity is reinforced visually by the repetition of words and fragments across the text, "chaining" all of the elements together.[1]

As rhetors argue for a hierarchy of cell types and strengthen their argument through repetition, they also create and amplify uncertainty and ambiguity about the specific levels of potency and the placement of cells within the hierarchy. Perelman and Olbrechts-Tyteca (1969) note that the use of an idea in an argument influences the level of ambiguity associated with it: Clarifying one element of an idea automatically obscures other elements. Kenneth Burke (1969a) argues that this ambiguity is an inevitable part of any system of symbols: "We take it for granted that, insofar as men cannot themselves create the universe, there must remain something essentially enigmatic about the problem of motives, and that this underlying enigma will manifest itself in inevitable ambiguities and inconsistencies" (p. xviii). Ambiguity is an essential part of the discourse and symbols we use to explain the world, and if ambiguity exists in all discourse, it will be especially apparent in scientific discourse, where "scientists must find ways of talking about what they do not know—about that which they as yet have only glimpses, guesses, speculations" (Keller, 2002, p. 118). Yet, this ambiguity is no mere stumbling block for scientists. Ambiguity is a productive force in science: Explanation often "depends on productive use of the cognitive tensions generated by multiple meanings, by ambiguity" (Keller, 2002, p. 117).

According to Keller (2002), ambiguity acts as a productive force in four ways. First, it can impel scientists to uncover clear and literal descriptions of phenomena that had previously been described in vague terms. Second, imprecision and ambiguity can fill in the gaps in scientific explanations. When scientists lack the abilities, tools, or methods to answer certain questions, ambiguous answers can serve as stopgap explanations. Third, in addition to acting as a stopgap, ambiguous concepts provide a resource for explanation as well as a means of concealing issues that cannot be currently answered. According to Keller, a certain level of ambiguity in key concepts can unify multiple disparate ways of addressing phenomena and provide a framework for generating and justifying new hypotheses for research. By maintaining certain forms of ambiguity, scientists can maintain a powerful engine for hypothesis generation and discovery. Fourth, ambiguity is necessary for scientists to speak across differing experimental programs and contexts. Ambiguity is necessary for communication. Language cannot be tied to the particular in an absolute fashion if it is to allow us to draw connections between different events—to see the similarity between events that seem prima facie dissimilar—which is a goal not only of everyday language use, but of scientific explanation as well.

Scientific Ranking of Stem Cell Types

Scientists studying stem cells try to organize and rank the types of cells they encounter. That ranking works through a hierarchy in which the cell types are organized by their association with a hierarchy of potency terms. The use of the hierarchy automatically establishes a similarity between cell types and implies that the differences between them are differences of degree, not kind. Thus, the use of the argument from hierarchy *creates* a relationship between the types of cells, which otherwise come from different organs in the human body and from human bodies at radically different stages of development. These differences in potency degree provide the basis for arguing that pluripotent ES cells will help scientists reach their research and therapeutic goals more effectively than adult stem cells, yet the ambiguities that inhere in the hierarchy also provide the basis for arguments opposing this claim.

The Potency Hierarchy

The levels of the potency hierarchy consist of two elements: a prefix denoting the extent of the potency (toti-, pluri-, and multi-, in decreasing order of strength) and the word "potency" itself, which is repeated at each level. The term "potent" first appeared in the English language almost 500 years ago and was originally used to refer to power. Its use then expanded to cover the idea of the "power of development" and the "power" of male sexuality (Pearsall & Trumbull, 2002). In scientific usage, "potency" usually refers to the power of a cell to differentiate into many different types of cells. In a parallel move, Nichols (2001) defines potency as "flexibility"—cells have a capacity to twist and shape themselves into different cell types.

The potency hierarchy is divided into a series of steps through the use of prefixes denoting different levels of power. The combination of prefix and root word establishes similarity and difference: Cells are similar in that they have power, in this case power to differentiate, but they differ in the degree to which they hold that power. The highest level of the potency hierarchy is totipotency, which refers to a cell's ability to become all the cells of the fetus, as well as the trophectoderm, the cells that form the placenta (Gage, 2000; Nichols, 2001; Smith, 2001; Thomson et al., 1995). The next level, pluripotency, refers to cells with the ability to become all types of cells, except those of the placenta (Gage, 2000; Nichols, 2001; Smith, 2001). After pluripotency, scientists place multipotency. Multipotency is less clearly defined throughout the literature (Gage, 2000).[2] After multipotency comes the use of specific potency terms like tripotent (Bjornson, Rietze, Reynolds, Magli, & Vescovi, 1999), bipotent (Mitaka, 2001; Theise et al., 2000), and unipotent (Slack, 2000), where the prefix indicates the exact number of differentiated progeny a cell can produce.[3]

Researchers create this hierarchy of potencies both discursively and visually through the text of their published articles, tables that offer brief textual definitions, and charts and figures combining visual and textual elements (Daniels, Dart, Tuft, & Khaw, 2001; Gage, 2000; Nichols, 2001; Watt, 2001; Watt & Hogan, 2000; Weissman, 2000a, 2000b; Weissman, Anderson, & Gage, 2001). The creation of this hierarchy links the different cell types together, transforming what could potentially be a difference in *kind* into a difference of *degree*. Some researchers have questioned whether the same molecular and genetic signals produce totipotency, pluripotency, and multipotency (Gage, 2000; Smith, 2001; Verfaillie, 2002; Wulf, Jackson, & Goodell, 2001). According to these researchers, it is not clear whether the same mechanisms work to create "potency" in all cells and how this mechanism is altered to produce cells with varying degrees of potency. Yet, most researchers do not raise these questions for two reasons. First, a lack of experimental data means that scientists have no grounds to challenge the potency hierarchy and the genetic and molecular similarity between potency types that it assumes. Second, the use of repetition in the hierarchy lends rhetorical force to the belief that potency exists as a continuum. The various levels of the hierarchy are tied together through the use of "potency" in the naming of each level. The repetition of the word creates a discursive chain linking "toti*potency*" with "pluri*potency*" and "multi*potency*." With the hierarchy, all types of stem cells are defined in terms of the same quality. This similarity increases the explanatory power of any set of scientific experiments: Work on pluripotent ES cells can be used as the basis for universal claims about all types of cell types, with appropriate reductions in the supposed power of the cells to reflect diminished levels of potency. Ultimately, the hierarchy becomes a reasonable hypothesis that is congruent with the available information while also extending beyond that information to provide a powerful explanatory framework for ongoing stem cell research.

The Hierarchy of Cell Types

Potency is the basis for the hierarchy of cell types. In scientific rhetoric concerning stem cells, three levels of the hierarchy are most important: "totipotent" fertilized eggs, "pluripotent" ES cells, and "multipotent" adult stem cells or progenitor cells. Totipotent cells—fertilized eggs—are unavailable for research for ethical and legal reasons, but "totipotency" represents an ideal in scientific rhetoric about stem cells. An understanding of the "total power" of fertilized eggs would help scientists understand the earliest stages of mammalian development—one of the scientific applications of stem cells. Harnessing totipotency would allow scientists to create all the cell types in the human body, which means that scientists could create many different types of cells for pharmaceutical and medical applications. Totipotency is associated with cells capable of becoming any other type of cell. These are fertilized eggs or "reprogrammed" cells that can be implanted in the uterus to produce a clone (Bjornson et al., 1999; Gage, 2000).[4]

Pluripotency is usually associated with ES cells. This association appears in three different forms. First, some review articles make the entire hierarchy of potency and the associated cell types explicit, thus allowing audiences to perceive the entire range of power and cell types and the placement of ES cells on that continuum (Gage, 2000; Nichols, 2001; Watt & Hogan, 2000). Second, many other articles make the connection between pluripotency and ES cells apparent and provide one other level of the hierarchy as a point of contrast: Some researchers contrast pluripotent ES cells with totipotent cells like the fertilized egg (Tada, Takahama, Abe, Nakatsuji, & Tada, 2001; Thomson et al., 1998; Thomson et al., 1995), while others contrast ES cells with the weaker multipotent adult stem cells (Pittenger et al., 1999; Smith, 2001; Verfaillie, 2002; Wulf et al., 2001). Finally, some authors describe ES cells as pluripotent without providing a point of contrast, making the description either an assertion or an enthymeme depending on the knowledge and other discursive fragments audiences can bring to bear on the text (Amit et al., 2000; Evans & Kaufman, 1981; Martin, 1981; Nichols et al., 1998; Thomson & Odorico, 2000).

The next level, multipotency, is usually associated with adult stem cells. The most explicit presentations of the argument from hierarchy make this association (Gage, 2000; Nichols, 2001; Watt, 2001; Watt & Hogan, 2000). It also appears in a number of other review and research articles that focus primarily on tissue-specific stem cells from adults, like epithelial, hematopoietic, and mesenchymal stem cells (Ferrari et al., 1998; Goodell, Brose, Paradis, Conner, & Mulligan, 1996; Jackson et al., 2001; Lagasse et al., 2000; Pittenger et al., 1999; Slack, 2000; Springer, Brazelton, & Blau, 2001; Weissman et al., 2001). In addition to this association, "multipotent" is also used to describe progenitor cells—a level of cells usually described as intermediaries between stem cells and the differentiated cells that constitute the body. Weissman (2000a) and Jackson et al. (2001) use "multipotent" to refer to both stem cells and progenitor cells, and researchers from the University of Minnesota isolated a group of cells they describe as multipotent adult progenitor cells (MAPCs) (Reyes et al., 2002; Reyes & Verfaillie, 2001; Schwartz et al., 2002; Verfaillie, 2002). Even with this overlap of terminology, researchers still describe progenitor cells as a lower level of the hierarchy, just a step above those cells that have no capacity for differentiation.

The hierarchy of potency terms and cell types provides a discursive basis for claims about which types of stem cells will provide the best route to the applications valued by scientists. After examining the research on both adult and ES cells, Watt and Hogan (2000) conclude their review with the following observation: "[Studies of ES cells] hold great promise not only for unexpected insights into biology but ultimately for the alleviation of human suffering" (p. 1430). For Watt and Hogan, ES cells will help scientists achieve two of the purposes of stem cell research. In a similar move, Gage (2000) identifies ES cells as the type of cells most likely to be used for clinical and commercial applications (p. 1434). After contrasting embryonic and adult stem cells, Nichols (2001) says, "stem cells derived from embryos are likely to prove to be the most efficient route for tissue replacement therapy" (p. R503), and Smith (2001) claims that it will be more difficult to transform adult stem cells into cell-replacement therapies than it would using ES cells. These arguments develop out of the hierarchical placement of embryonic and adult stem cells, and they tie the use of that hierarchy to the potential applications of stem cell research. Since ES cells are more potent—able to create more types of cells—researchers can do more research and produce more cell-replacement therapies with them than they could with the more limited adult stem cells.

Ambiguity in the Scientific Argument from Hierarchy

The creation of a potency hierarchy provides in part the basis for claims that ES cells will be the best means of developing hoped-for applications, but the very use of the hierarchy also creates the opportunity for counterclaims that adult stem cells have similar potency. The ambiguity provides the basis for counterclaims that adult stem cells are just as efficacious as ES cells, while also having the benefit of sidestepping ethical issues surrounding the use of embryonic tissue. The ambiguity in the hierarchy takes two forms: *semantic ambiguities* involving how levels of potency are defined and *categorical ambiguities* involving which cell types belong to a given category.

First, there is a semantic ambiguity in the prefixes used to denote levels of power, and this semantic ambiguity has the potential to destabilize the hierarchy of cell types. This semantic ambiguity arises between the terms "pluripotency" and "multipotency." According to *The Oxford English Dictionary* (Pearsall & Trumbull, 2002), the prefix "pluri-" means "much" or "several," and the prefix "multi-" means "many" or "much." Neither prefix provides an exact amount: It is not clear how many objects must come together to count as "much," and it is not clear in the scientific literature how many different cell types must be produced by a stem cell to count as multipotency or pluripotency. The two prefixes overlap, and terms into which they are incorporated share that overlap and ambiguity in meaning. Both terms refer to an uncertain degree of power or potency, and it is only the assertion by scientists that defines pluripotency as a greater degree of power.

While ambiguity exists between the two terms, there is a degree of semantic ambiguity contained within the term "multipotency." Scientists attribute a broad range of potency to "multipotency." Many scientists specify a particular number of different cell types that can be produced, although none of these exact definitions are taken up outside of the article that introduces them. Jonathan Slack (2000) defines "multipotency" as the ability to produce four unique types of cells, but then he also claims that many adult stem cells are normally unipotent (see also Daniels et al., 2001). Bjornson et al. (1999) identify neural stem cells as "tripotent"—as being able to produce three different types of cells. Mitaka (2001) and Theise et al. (2000) describe liver stem cells as being bipotent. In each case, the authors also describe the cells they discuss as multipotent, thus temporarily narrowing the definition of "multipotency," sometimes to the point that it refers to producing one new type of cell only.

The semantic ambiguity is amplified by categorical ambiguities involving the attribution of specific levels of power to different types of cells. These categorical ambiguities appear in relation to two groups of cells: committed progenitor cells and hematopoietic stem cells. According to the argument from hierarchy, progenitor cells are the immediate offspring of stem cells that lead to the final specific cell types, such as liver cell, neuron, and so on, but their potency—while marked both as less than that of adult stem cells and as less than that identified by the category "multipotency"—has been described by some scientists as greater than the amount specified for many adult stem cells. Weissman (2000a; 2000b; Weissman et al., 2001) describes progenitor cells that can produce two to four different progeny. Researchers at the University of Minnesota described MAPCs—*multipotent* adult progenitor cells—that reportedly can become multiple cell types from different embryonic layers, a capacity that is supposedly beyond the power of progenitor cells and most adult stem cells (Reyes et al.,

2002; Schwartz et al., 2002). According to Reyes and Verfaillie (2001), multipotent adult progenitor cells can be differentiated into *11* different cell types, more than almost all adult stem cell types. The existence of these extremely powerful multipotent progenitors disturbs the ranking that places merely tri- or bipotent adult stem cells above them.

In addition to the ambiguity in the placement of progenitor cells, the description of adult stem cells, especially hematopoietic stem cells, by some scientists troubles their placement in the hierarchy. Scientists reviewing work on adult stem cells observe that the research raises questions about the degree of potency they exhibit. Wulf et al. (2001) observe, "Still an open question is whether there are somatic [adult] stem cells with true pluripotency" (p. 1368). Verfaillie (2002) remarks, "Although the discussion above indicates that stem cell plasticity is not proven, there is sufficient evidence to warrant continued efforts to prove or disprove that some adult stem cells might be more pluripotent" (p. 507). The interpretation of the experimental evidence raises questions for these scientists about the power of some adult stem cells: Their categorization—their location in the hierarchy of cell types—is ambiguous. That categorical ambiguity is amplified by semantic ambiguity in some discussions of hematopoietic stem cells. In reporting their experimental findings that the blood-forming hematopoietic stem cells (HSCs) produce cells of the liver, Lagasse and colleagues (2000) say, "If resident bone marrow HSCs can form a variety of cell types, they may be more multipotent than the phrase 'pluripotent hematopoietic stem cell' indicates" (p. 1232). Here, the normal ranking of the two terms is troubled, if not completely reversed. The categorical ambiguity in the placement of hematopoietic stem cells on the hierarchy augments the semantic ambiguity: The meaning of the categories used to organize cell types becomes troubled just as the attempt to categorize one type of cell is troubled.

These categorical and semantic ambiguities do three things. First, these ambiguities amplify the assumptions built into the hierarchy. The hierarchy assumes an underlying similarity—a generic and uniform "potency"—between cell types, specifically that differentiation, which potency measures, works in a similar fashion in all cells. This claim is implicit in the hierarchy, although scientists explicitly note that the molecular mechanisms of differentiation are not clearly understood and may differ between different types of stem and progenitor cells (Gage, 2000; Smith, 2001). This assumption, built into the hierarchy and amplified by its ambiguity, acts as a stopgap explanation covering the inability of scientists at that specific point in time to fully explain stem cell differentiation. By treating all stem cells and progenitor cells as performing the same function with various degrees of success, the argument from hierarchy (and its attendant ambiguities) reduces the number of intractable issues facing scientists at any one point. More recently, scientists have begun to identify genetic mechanisms for stem cell *pluripotency,* but they leave unaddressed the mechanisms shaping other levels of potency (Gearhart, Pashos, & Prasad, 2007; Lengner et al., 2007; Takahashi & Yamanaka, 2006).

Second, the ambiguities in the argument from hierarchy allow scientists to speak across different research domains. While the work on ES cells uses different molecular markers and slightly different techniques from those used on adult stem cells, the ambiguity in language allows scientists to bridge the different laboratory and experimental contexts that produced the results they report. Third, the ambiguities surrounding adult stem cell potency are generative of more research. As described above, scientists note the lack of definitive evidence, but claim that sufficient evidence exists to continue research in these areas. Often, this appeal to continued research is amplified by linking research on adult stem cells to the possibility of medical applications. In the conclusion of their review article, Wulf and colleagues (2001) note, "The recent findings in stem cell biology reviewed here, together with their projected therapeutic implications in transplantation medicine, justify our optimistic attention to the future in somatic [adult] stem cells" (p. 1368; see also Mezey, Chandross, Harta, Maki, & McKercher, 2000; Watt & Hogan, 2000). Jackson, Mi, and Goodell (1999) also make this claim and implicitly refer to the moral objections individuals have with using ES cells: "If stem cells from adult tissues are generally found to have a broad potential to differentiate, it may not be necessary to use embryonic stem cells in some medical and experimental settings" (p. 14485). The possibility of greater potency in adult stem cells not only justifies their use in experimental and laboratory settings, but it also makes them an alternative to ES cells, which some people find morally objectionable (see also Wurmser & Gage, 2002).

Scientistic Idiom and Arguments from Hierarchy

Discourse in the public sphere also makes use of the argument from hierarchy. Like scientists, the public must organize the types of stem cells and adjudicate claims that different stem cell types will lead to the applications desired by the public. Scientistic uses of the hierarchy argument take four forms. The first two, which also appear in science, are a straightforward reading of the hierarchy that emphasizes the power of ES cells, and an emphasis on the hierarchy's ambiguities that undergirds claims that adult stem cells will be as effective as ES cells. The give-and-take of public debate leads to two additional rhetorical tactics: reaffirmations of the hierarchy that require an increased dependence on scientific rhetoric and ambivalent responses advocating both embryonic and adult stem cell research.

Defining "Potency" and Deploying the Hierarchy

To categorize stem cells and the relative power of each type, public rhetors first must establish the hierarchy of potency terms and cell types. This occurs during the earliest congressional testimony and newspaper coverage as well as in the NIH's 2001 report on stem cell research. Once components of the hierarchy circulate in the public sphere, rhetors can then deploy claims depending on it, or the ambiguities within it can be recognized and exploited. Rhetors establish the hierarchy in two ways. First, many scientists present a narrative of development that associates the greatest potency with the earliest stages of life. Second, non-scientists stipulate definitions for some of the key potency terms in the hierarchy.

Scientific rhetors often use a developmental narrative that strengthens the hierarchy by adding temporal priority to the logical and categorical priorities already built into it. The order within which a story is told can be used to strengthen a "timeless" categorical or logical organization. Some temporal orderings are subtle. For example, Thomas Okarma of Geron Corporation notes, "hES [human Embryonic Stem] cells can form virtually any cell in the body. Specifically they have the potential to form derivatives of all three cellular layers. . . . Other later stage human stem cells have only a limited capability to form certain cell types such as blood cells (CD34+ stem cells) or connective tissues (mesenchymal stem cells)" (*Stem Cell Research*, 1999, p. 54). The use of "later" creates a temporal order that links the potency of the two categories of stem cells to temporal "stages" of the human body.

The most explicit use of development in the deployment of the hierarchy occurs in the prepared testimony of Drs. Allen Spiegel and Gerald Fischbach in April 2000:

> [Stem cells] are best described in the context of normal human development. When a sperm fertilizes an egg, the product is a single cell that has the potential to form an entire organism. This fertilized egg is a totipotent stem cell, which has the potential to develop into a complete organism. In the first hours and days after fertilization, this cell begins to divide into identical totipotent stem cells. Then, approximately four days after fertilization, these totipotent stem cells begin to specialize, forming a hollow sphere of cells called a blastocyst. One part of the blastocyst is a cluster of cells called the inner cell mass, which are the stem cells that will go on to form most of the cells and tissues of the human body. These are pluripo-

tent stem cells, which are different than totipotent stem cells. Pluripotent stem cells do not develop into a complete organism. (*Stem Cell Research, part 3,* 2000, p. 5)

The hierarchy of potencies and stem cell types appears here as an integral element of the story of human fetal development. Totipotency is tied to the fertilized egg and the earliest cells of the embryo. Pluripotency and ES cells are associated with the inner cell mass of the blastocyst, the next stage of embryonic development.[5] Each potency term and the associated cell type are tied to a specific stage in the story of development.

The prepared testimony of NIH director Harold Varmus adds the next stage of the story—the development of the embryos into a child and adult, and the concomitant rise of more limited adult stem cells:

> During fetal development, pluripotent stem cells become even more committed, i.e., they have the capacity to form only one or a few different kinds of cells. For example, hematopoietic stem cells can form all the blood cells, but no other tissue types. The adult human being continues to harbor many types of stem cells responsible for the body's ability to repair some but not all tissues. Stem cells that permit new skin growth and renewal of blood cells are two examples. (*Stem Cell Research,* 1999, p. 9)

With the move from embryo through fetus to adult, the stem cells become more restricted in their potency, continuing the narrative trend that temporal distance from conception results in diminished power.

The NIH report *Stem Cells: Scientific Progress and Future Research Directions* also deploys the developmental narrative, and it likewise employs a didactic tone when describing three stages of development and the related levels of potency— totipotency, pluripotency, and unipotency. At each stage of development and potency, the report provides an etymology of the Latin prefix used with the term, thus emphasizing the report's nature as a didactic text meant to inform the public and the government about the state of stem cell research. The report begins by describing totipotency and tying it to the fertilized egg. Like the narratives in congressional testimony, it then moves to pluripotency:

> Most scientists use the term pluripotent to describe stem cells that can give rise to cells derived from all three embryonic germ layers—mesoderm, endoderm, and ectoderm. These three germ layers are the embryonic source of all cells of the body . . . . "Pluri"—derived from the Latin *plures*—means several or many. Thus, pluripotent cells have the potential to give rise to

any type of cell, a property observed in the natural course of embryonic development and under certain laboratory conditions. (National Institutes of Health, 2001, p. 1)

While not explicitly naming ES cells, the emphasis on "the natural course of embryonic development" ties pluripotency to stem cells derived from the embryo. Finally, the report describes unipotent cells: "Unipotent stem cell, a term that is usually applied to a cell in adult organisms, means that the cells in question are capable of differentiating along only one lineage" (p. 1). With unipotency, one reaches the end of the developmental narrative and the bottom of the combined hierarchy of potency and cell type.

Nonscientists in congressional discourse stipulate loosely etymological definitions of terms from the hierarchy, especially "pluripotency." Richard Doerflinger defines pluripotency as "producing a wide array of different cells and tissues" (*Human Cloning,* 2001, p. 87). This definition derives from the understanding of potency as developmental power and the definition of "pluri-" as many. Other rhetors continue this trend but tie pluripotency to specific cell types. During a hearing panel on patent issues, Q. Todd Dickinson says, "Some stem cells are 'pluripotent' cell lines, meaning they can be made to develop into a variety of different specialized cells" (*Stem Cell Research,* 1999, p. 89). The commonsense definition of "pluripotency" becomes linked to specific stem cell lines, and although Dickinson does not specifically mention human ES cells, his entire testimony and the session during which it is given deals solely with the commercial and medical implications of isolating human ES cells.

Newspapers also stipulate the definitions of one or two potency terms.[6] Cleveland's *Plain Dealer* presents its definitions within a didactic and developmental narrative. After noting "we begin life as a single cell," the article describes the fertilized egg: "That first cell is called 'totipotent,' meaning it can give rise to all the embryo's tissues and to the membranes and tissues required to support its development in the womb, such as the placenta" (Haybron, 1999). Shortly after this description appears, the article describes the inner cell mass of an early-stage embryo: "These cells are termed 'pluripotent,' meaning they can give rise to most kinds of cells but are already too specialized to produce a complete, viable embryo" (Haybron, 1999). *The Omaha World Herald* notes that ES cells are "'pluripotent,' which means they can generate any type of cell in the body," and "adult stem cells are thought to be 'multipotent,' which means they can produce only limited cell types" (Olson, 2000e). The didactic tone maintains the general tenor of science journalism (Bucchi, 1998; Fahnestock, 1993), thus creating a scientistic aura. In emulating the didactic tone familiar to science journalism, newspaper coverage stipulates the meaning of these terms but does not provide an etymological definition or an exact count of the cell types produced. Rather, comparisons between terms provide additional meaning to these general definitions: Placing "totipotency" and "pluripotency," or "pluripotency" and "multipotency," near each other creates a context for better understanding the comparative levels of power described as well as placing the types of stem cells at differing levels of a hierarchy shaped by potency.

As the public debate about ES cell research heats up between mid-2000 and August 2001, news coverage shifts from an informative, or educational, approach in which the terminology and scientific complexities are explained to a description of the ethical and political field of debate, thus switching from approaches that favor a scientistic idiom to ones that frame the issues in an increasingly Manichean idiom of science and its political supporters versus religion and its political supporters. As a result, the relative potency of ES cells in relation to adult stem cells is increasingly asserted. *The St. Louis Post-Dispatch* claims, "It has long been believed that only embryonic stem cells—which are removed from the unborn—have the ability to develop into any other cell type in the body" ("Research Indicates," 2000). *The Omaha World-Herald* declares, "Scientists aren't sure that adult stem cells have as much versatility or potential for medical breakthroughs as the stem cells from embryos left over from in-vitro fertilization" (Olson, 2000a). On the night President Bush announced his funding decision, CBS's Elizabeth Kaledin said, "Stem cells can be harvested from a variety of places. . . . But it's the cells taken from frozen embryos that scientists say hold the most promise" ("Embryonic Stem Cell Research," 2001). In early September 2001, *USA Today* noted, "Stem cells extracted from human embryos are the most promising because they're so young that they can be turned into any cells in the human body. . . . Adult and infant stem cells aren't as exciting since they can only be used to regenerate the tissue they come from" (Krantz, 2001). In these articles, the relative potency of each cell type is treated as an argument in favor of ES cell research, which is coordinated with the other issues raised in favor of ES cell research and balanced against the concerns raised by opponents.

Although it appears rarely, there is one final use of the hierarchy. It overemphasizes the potency of ES cells to portray them as dangerous and medically unsafe. According to Dr. David Prentice, ES cells are more than pluripotent, and this near-totipotency is dangerous: "Although human embryonic stem cells may exhibit impressive plasticity due to their potency, this plasticity has been proven to be a double-edged sword, as embryonic stem cells have been difficult to control in laboratories" (*Opportunities and Advancements,* 2001, p. 123). Here the association of ES cells with pluripotency is described as "plasticity," but greater potency now has dubious value. Prentice claims that ES cells may become many things and that scientists find this ability almost impossible to control. ES cells become a Frankenstein monster in a Petri dish—a technological terror that could wreak havoc if it were to escape the laboratory and enter the hospital. The dangers of ES cells are also emphasized by Dr. Maria Michejda, who contrasts the out-of-control ES cells with the "tamer," less potent fetal stem cells obtained from spontaneous abortions: "Fetal stem cells have most of the properties of embryonic stem cells but do not exhibit the uncontrolled replication that is a characteristic of embryonic cells, which leads to teratomas, malignancies and chromosomal mosaicism upon transplantation" (*Cloning,* 2002, p. 23). According to Michejda, ES cells cause cancer—teratomas and malignancies—or create chimeras, individuals who have a mosaic of DNA from multiple source animals. The threat of cancer is meant to arouse fear, and the concern about mosaicism, which leads to chimeric individuals, replays fears embodied in the Frankenstein myth of half-human monsters running amok (Rushing & Frentz, 1989).

These statements recognize the placement of ES cells in relation to adult stem cells in the hierarchy argument: ES cells are more potent than adult stem cells. This dystopian vision of ES cell application becomes a viable depiction of their applications because the exact form applications of ES cells will take is unknown. This provides the rhetors in this debate considerable leeway in creating a possible future upon which they can base their arguments. Furthermore, opponents invent this dystopian vision of the future by drawing from a narrow and specific component of the past: the earliest research establishing the existence of ES cells in mice and humans. This research involved the creation of teratomas and mouse chimeras (Evans & Kaufman, 1981; Martin, 1981; National Institutes of Health, 2001; Thomson et al., 1998; Thomson et al., 1995). In order to establish that the cells they had isolated were in fact ES cells able to produce all three germ layers of the early embryo, researchers would inject the stem cells under the skin of mice whose immune systems were incapable of rejecting foreign tissue. They would then remove the resulting tumor and examine it under a microscope to determine what types of tissues had developed. Another test for stem cells involved injecting them into developing mouse embryos. If the embryo successfully developed, scientists could employ a number of visual and genetic tests to determine if the putative stem cells had successfully differentiated and been incorporated into the new animal, a mouse chimera or hybrid. The picture of dangerous and out-of-control ES cells wreaking havoc in unsuspecting patients portrays the early research on ES cells *as the actual medical application of ES cells.* Yet, as the NIH report on stem cell research notes, "The lines of unaltered human embryonic stem cells that exist will not be suitable for direct use in patients. These cells will need to be differentiated or otherwise modified before they can be used clinically" (National Institutes of Health, 2001, p. ES-5). Injecting any form of stem cell directly into an individual is a dangerous and risky practice. Scientists do not plan to create teratomas in individuals by randomly injecting stem cells into unsuspecting patients.

Deploying Ambiguity

Along with the deployment of the potency-based hierarchy, the ambiguities resulting from that hierarchy are also available for use. Critics use the ambiguities, along with the concept of adult stem cell plasticity, to discredit ES cell research and to claim that adult stem cells have a level of potency equal to, and possibly greater than, ES cells. Claims of greater or equivalent potency function as an enthymeme: Potent cells can become many cell types; degree of differentiation (potency) increases the likelihood of medical application; therefore, greater potency means a greater number of applications. Rhetors often pair the claim of equivalent potency with claims about the existing medical applications of adult stem cells or the lack of existing medical applications for ES cells.

Rhetors often use the word "versatility" to refer to the potency of adult stem cells. "Versatility" is a synonym for "flexibility," the term used by some scientists to define pluripotency (Nichols, 2001), and opponents tie the term directly to use or application. For example, Rep. Jay Dickey (R–AR) claims, "Numerous reports over just the last few months have shown remarkable discoveries about the versatility and possible uses of stem cells found in adults" (*Stem Cell Research, part 2,* 1999, p. 10). Dr. Micheline Mathews-Roth links her claim about adult stem cell "versatility" to the accusation that the NIH ignored the phenomenon: "The Guidelines [established in 2000, but never put into practice] . . . seem to ignore the mounting evidence in the current scientific literature of the versatility of adult stem cells" (*Stem Cell Research, part 3,* 2000, p. 71). Another approach to arguing that adult stem cells have equivalent potency or "versatility" treats adult stem cells as a collective whole. According to Judy Norsigian, founder of Boston Women's Health Book Collective, "It turns out that taken as a collective, the population of adult stem cells has as wide a potential as embryo stem cells" (*Dangers of Cloning,* 2002, p. 34). This perspective argues that while any single type of adult stem cell might not have as much potency as ES cells, all adult stem cells, taken as a whole, have potency equivalent to ES cells.

In newspapers, many discussions of equivalent potency appear in reports about new scientific findings. For example, news coverage of Bjornson and colleagues' (1999) report that neural stem cells could become cells found in blood led to journalistic observations about adult stem cell plasticity. *The Seattle Times* quoted a local researcher who noted, "The stem cells are more plastic (changeable) than anyone ever thought" (King, 1999). The first author of the study, Christopher Bjornson, observes, "The mature stem cells are a lot more plastic than we imagined" (Associated Press, 1999). Stem cells from adults are more plastic and therefore more potent than previously believed. While that potency is not directly compared to the power of ES cells, the implication is that these cells are similar to their embryonic counterparts.

Additionally, the structure of newspaper articles and the journalistic desire for objectivity produce ambiguity about the potency of each stem cell type. *The Milwaukee Journal Sentinel's* report on the Vatican's condemnation of ES cell research notes, "In some instances, adult cells have been shown to have developmental capacities similar to those of embryonic cells—but, say McKay and Wisconsin researchers, those cells often stop dividing early, and their potential could be limited" (Schubert & Fauber, 2000b). *The Washington Post* at one point claims, "So far, human embryo and fetal cells have shown unparalleled potential to rejuvenate aging tissues and organs," and later remarks on "growing evidence that adult cells have much, if not all, the therapeutic potential once thought unique to embryo cells" (Weiss, 2000c). Within the space of a paragraph, the Minneapolis *Star Tribune* goes from observing that "recent research has shown that the adult stem cells are more flexible than previously believed" to reporting that the NIH believes "adult cells may not have the versatility of embryonic cells" (Schmickle, 2000a). These articles follow the journalistic standard of presenting both sides of an issue and present claims about each type of stem cell without providing a judgment or conclusion about the merits of these claims. Unfortunately, the articles also fail to provide enough information for readers to construct their own judgments about the respective claims.

Ambiguity allows for claims that adult stem cells have sufficient potency or plasticity to be considered for the same uses as ES cells. The political uses of ambiguity examined so far work to undo the previous placement of adult stem cells into a less potent category, and while some newspaper coverage leads to similar results, many newspaper reports do not provide a means of adjudicating the various claims. Some rhetors try to use the ambiguity in the hierarchy to go beyond generating claims about equivalent potency: They try to tie claims about adult stem cell potency to attacks on the value of ES cells. Richard Doerflinger claims, "Adult stem cells may be more versatile than was once thought [and, therefore,] offer the promise that embryonic stem cells may simply be irrelevant to medical progress" (*Stem Cell Research,* 1999, p. 134). Adult stem cell versatility "promises" to make ES cells irrelevant and unnecessary. Dr. Frank Young advances a similar claim about adult stem cells: "Recent studies have demonstrated that these cells might be a suitable substitute for ES and EG [embryonic germ] cells" (*Stem Cell Research, part 2,* 1999, p. 6). These claims operate scientifically to create a "fact" about adult stem cells—that they have sufficient potency to create medical applications—which can then be incorporated into broader objections to ES cell research. While these objections are typically grounded in religious and ethical concerns, that aspect of the argument is muted.

While discourse in congressional hearings is coy about the religious basis for arguments supporting adult stem cells over ES cells, those religious and ethical components become explicit in some news coverage. *The Pittsburgh Post-Gazette*'s article on stem cell research conducted at the University of Pittsburgh reports, "But a string of recent discoveries has shown that even these adult stem cells have the capability to produce a variety of cell types, perhaps simply by changing their environment or the chemical signals sent to them. If so, the controversial use of stem cells from aborted fetuses may prove unnecessary" (Srikameswaran, 1999a).[7] In 2000, *The Omaha World Herald* reports claims that adult stem cell research "essentially circumvents all the ethical concerns" (Olson, 2000b), and *The Boston Globe* in 2002 asserts adult stem cells "have equivalent healing potential without the ethical baggage" (Mishra, 2002).

Finally, some rhetors tie the claim of adult stem cell potency to an argument that the therapeutic potential of ES cells is an uncertain path, at best, to relieving suffering. An extended version of this claim appears in Rep. Mark Souder's (R–IN) opening statement to the House Committee on Government Reform's subcommittee on criminal justice's hearing on ES cell research:

> "Adult" stem cells capable of transforming into countless cells and tissue types have been located throughout the human body, including in the brain, muscles, blood, placentas and even in fat. Researchers have only begun to unlock the potential of these adult stem cells.
>
> Stem cells from fat have been transformed into cartilage, muscle and bone. Adult bone marrow stem cells have been transformed into muscle, cardiac tissues, neural cells, liver, bone, cartilage and fat. And just this May, researchers announced that they had identified an adult cell that appears capable of becoming virtually any cell in the body.
>
> Contrary to the impressions created by advocates for embryonic stem cell research, the potential of such cells remains entirely speculative, because embryonic stem cells have never been successfully used in clinical applications with human patients. Lost in the debate is the fact that all of the clinically successful human applications of stem cells to date have been conducted with adult stem cells. . . . There is no reason, therefore, to believe that adult stem cells do not have the same—if not greater—potential than stem cells derived from embryos. (*Opportunities and Advancements,* 2001, p. 2)

The argument begins with a general claim about adult stem cell versatility—they can become "countless" tissue types. Souder then enumerates several different adult stem cell types and the tissues into which they differentiate: With each sentence, the number of cell types that adult stem cells can produce increases, thus creating the perception of substantial degrees of potency. After establishing this broad potency in adult stem cells and contrasting the extant uses of bone marrow stem cells to the potential uses of ES cells, Souder affirms that adult stem cells have as much potency as, if not more than, ES cells.

Claims that adult stem cells have greater medical utility than ES cells combine a broad range of discursive fragments, definitions, and lines of argument circulating in the scientific and public spheres. First, Souder draws from reports of recent scientific findings, touted in both journalistic and scientific venues, to define adult stem cells as having potency equal to ES cells. Souder is legitimately using scientific research reports from trusted publication venues like *Science* to make his claim. Scientific objections to the adult stem cell research he references had not yet been published, and at this point, they had only been circulated at scientific meetings and by a few scientists testifying at congressional hearings. Second, these claims reflect the fact that hematopoietic adult stem cells, which are the cells in bone marrow that replenish the blood supply and reconstitute the immune system, had been in medical use for decades. Yet, public discussion of these clinical uses in the stem cell debate deflects attention from two issues. First, ES cells might produce therapies for diseases that currently have no cure. Reconstituting the immune system after chemotherapy, which occurs with hematopoietic stem cells in bone marrow transplants, is a far cry from cures for Alzheimer's disease, Parkinson's disease, and diabetes, which are the cures promised by ES cell research. Second, the focus on hematopoietic stem cells obscures the fact that no population of adult stem cells besides hematopoietic stem cells is ready for clinical use (National Institutes of Health, 2001).

Responding to Ambiguity

Advocates of stem cell research do not let challenges grounded in the ambiguities of the hierarchy go unanswered. Some advocates merely reassert claims grounded in the hierarchical association of ES cells and "pluripotency." Dr. Douglas Melton says, "And I would simply like to say at this point that while adult stem cells have some similar properties, based on what we know today, adult stem cells do not have all the properties of embryonic stem cells" (*Stem Cell Research,* 2001, p. 59). Dr. Paul Berg claims, "Every scientific review of the therapeutic opportunities afforded by adult-derived and embryonic stem cells has concluded that embryonic stem cells are far more versatile for medical therapies" (*Dangers of Cloning,* 2002, p. 46). Melton asserts that the two categories are different but leaves the difference unspecified. Berg borrows opponents' use of "versatility" to describe the difference between adult stem and ES cells, and he explicitly ties it to medical therapies, while justifying this claim with a reference to scientific reviews of stem cell research. Both claims depend on the authority of science—either embodied by the speaker or found in the existence of scientific literature—for their validity.

Melton's and Berg's comments leave the debate about defining stem cell potency and the relative merits of each cell type at a stalemate: Each side repeats its previous positions without being able to move the debate beyond this point of contention. Some proponents try to shift the argument in favor of ES cell research by linking ES cell pluripotency to some other discursive fragment previously used to define "stem cell." Scientific rhetors incorporate fragments circulating primarily in scientific forums. Advanced Cell Technology's Michael West plays on the fact that ES cell precursors in the embryo build all the tissues of the body in order to claim that ES cells are better than adult stem cells: "The embryonic stem cell can self-assemble into a complex tissue given the right circumstances. It can actually form intestine and other kidney tissue and other important tissues—we've never seen this before in the history of medicine" (*Cloning,* 2001, p. 14). ES cells do more than become the components of various tissues; they have the capacity to assemble those cells into the proper order or configuration necessary to build viable tissue and organs.

Other rhetors reemphasize the ES cell's capacity for "self-renewal" and link that capacity to "pluripotency." Drs. Spiegel and Fischbach argue: "Pluripotent and adult stem cells are not qualitatively alike. Pluripotent stem cells have truly amazing abilities to self-renew and to form many different cell types, even complex tissues, but in contrast the full potential of adult stem cells is uncertain, and, in fact, there is evidence to suggest they may be more limited. Unlike pluripotent stem cells, the adult stem cells may be able to divide only a limited number of times, which would limit their usefulness in the production of adequate numbers of well characterized cells for reliable therapies" (*Stem Cell Research, part 3,* 2000, p. 8). Self-renewal is equated with pluripotency. The qualities are treated as two sides of the same coin, and both qualities become the basis for arguing that ES cells will be more effective than adult stem cells in producing therapies. Lawrence Goldstein also uses the issue of self-renewal when he declares that stem cells from embryos, fetuses, and adults are qualitatively different: "It is far too early to know if adult stem cells have the same potential as embryonic stem cells, whether they can be harvested in sufficient quantities to treat or cure disease, and whether they can grow indefinitely as can ES cells" (*Stem Cell Research, part 3,* 2000, p. 46). Alongside the issue of "potential" or potency,

Goldstein raises two other issues: self-renewal and a practical concern whether enough adult cells can be harvested to cure diseases. Self-renewal, which had originally been downplayed in the shift from the scientific to the political arena, is reemphasized as a key capacity for medical applications as well as research applications.

Scientific rhetors respond to claims about the power of adult stem cells by reviving fragments of scientific rhetoric. Self-renewal is a key property used to define stem cells in science. It is important for science since its existence allows researchers to develop stable, long-lived groups of cells that can be used for multiple experiments, thus minimizing the need to keep isolating cells and also providing the grounds for comparing multiple experiments since they occurred with the same group of cells. Yet, the importance of self-renewal was diminished when the debate moved to the public sphere. By trying to revive the use of the term, scientists do two things. First, they provide an additional point of contrast between ES and adult stem cells: They argue that not only do scientists believe that ES cells have greater potency, but ES cells also have another important quality that adult stem cells lack. Second, the move not only reinforces the scientistic idiom in which the debate occurs, it treats scientific discourse as a more secure source of knowledge. Typically, the scientistic idiom borrows the discursive trappings of science—thus, the use of scientific terminology about potency—while remaining independent of the specific findings of science. Arguments must *appear* scientific even though the specific claims might extend beyond (or possibly contradict) scientific findings, but with claims that revive the use of "self-renewal," scientists try to reverse this process and make the debate hinge upon specific scientific findings. Scientists imply that the public should accept this definition of ES cells (that they are more potent *and* self-renewing) because these claims are vouchsafed by scientific practice.

Another strategy, and one used by rhetors with and without a scientific affiliation, is to turn to *kairos* and reemphasize the timeliness with which ES cells will lead to medical applications. For these rhetors, ES cells will produce medical applications quickly, in contrast to adult stem cells. According to Christopher Reeve, "If the government forces scientists [to] attempt to make adult stem cells behave like embryonic stem cells, they might waste five years or more and fail. In the meantime, hundreds of thousands will have died" (*Dangers of Cloning*, 2002, p. 18). Devoting time and resources to adult stem cell research will be a quixotic venture that will result in the loss of lives. Senator Orrin Hatch (R-UT) also emphasizes the *kairos* of ES cell research, but he frames it in terms of the respective "stages" of embryonic and adult stem cell research. During testimony following the publication of NIH's report on the state of stem cell research in 2001, Hatch stated,

While I am not a scientist, my preliminary reading of the report strongly suggests that embryonic stem cell research may have some substantial advantages over adult stem cells, at least at this stage of the research. . . . However, it is important to note what the NIH report does not say. It does not say that the promise of embryonic stem cell research obviates the need to pursue adult stem cell research. The report indicates that both embryonic and adult stem cell research hold great promise. I believe that both avenues should be zealously pursued. (*Stem Cells, 2001,* 2001, p. 12)

ES cells currently show more promise for producing medical applications. The stage at which that research exists places it closer to potential applications. Yet, Hatch notes, both avenues of research hold promise and should both be pursued "zealously"—the two avenues of research, despite the apparent advantage of embryonic over adult stem cells, complement one another in their "great promise" for future therapies.

The language of "time lost" from Reeve's testimony and Hatch's comments about the "stages" of research are combined in testimony by Richard O. Hynes, the president of the American Society for Cell Biology. Hynes says,

Critics argue that embryonic stem cell research is unnecessary because stem cells from adult tissues may be equally effective. I regret that this claim is ill-informed and misleading. Recent reports on adult stem cells are indeed encouraging, but this line of research is in its very early stages and far from definitive at this point. We know little about the availability of adult stem cells, their differentiation, or their potential for prolonged maintenance outside the body.

While we strongly support continued research on adult stem cells, it is far too early to conclude that they will be as effective in treating and preventing disease as embryonic stem cells seem certain to be. If we hold up progress on embryonic stem cells we may be very much at a loss in a few years [*sic*] time. (*Stem Cell Research, part 3,* 2000, p. 85)

Adult stem cell research is in its earliest stages, and claims that it could replace research on ES cells are ill informed. Hynes emphasizes that stopping ES cell research is untimely: Years of research could be lost in the potentially futile quest to determine if adult stem cells have potency equivalent to ES cells.

Reaffirmations of the hierarchy and its placement of cell types almost always appear in political discourse. At best, news discourse dimly reflects this reaffirmation. For example, *The San Francisco Chronicle* notes that ES cells "are still considered the benchmark against which all other cell types are measured" (Hall,

2000). New Orleans's *Times-Picayune* says, "Most researchers believe that embryonic stem cells retain a greater ability to transform into other cells of the body than do stem cells from other sources" (Treadway, 2002). While not a direct transcription of attempts to reaffirm the hierarchy of cell types, these claims reflect the continued emphasis, especially by scientists, on the greater power of ES cells, as well as the attempt by scientists to make public discourse comport with scientific discourse on ES cells. News discourses do not provide more space for reaffirmations since these reaffirmations do not provide any new material or novelty, making them less newsworthy; but this strategy regularly appears in political discourse because of the need to continually repeat and reinforce one's point of view in order to keep it in political circulation.

Agnosticism and Equivocation

A final response to the debate about stem cell potencies takes comments about the complementarity of adult and ES cells, like those made by Hatch and Hynes, to the point of equivocation. This argument treats neither adult nor ES cells as better than the other. The equivocation reflects the ambiguity and uncertainty about different cell types and concerns about the timeliness of federal funding and research programs. Equivocal responses appear less frequently than the other types of arguments comparing adult stem cells and ES cells, and for the most part, political uses of this equivocation appeared during the month immediately before and the two months after President Bush's decision on ES cell research. These equivocal statements, whether produced by nonscientists (who make the majority of these claims) or scientists, attempt to manage the relationship between scientific research and science policy. The equivocal statements recognize the "gap" between specific scientific findings and the scientistic idiom of public debate, and they usually widen that gap.

While opening a committee hearing on stem cells on July 18, 2001, Senator Tom Harkin (D-IA) claims, "Embryonic and adult stem cells are different and both present immense research opportunities for potential therapies. I think it would be irresponsible to wait for years to determine the potential of adult stem cells before studying the benefits of embryonic stem cells" (*Stem Cells, 2001*, 2001, p. 2). Although he argues here for continued study of ES cells, the basis for his argument is that ES cells *and* adult stem cells both represent promising routes to medical therapies. Waiting for science to determine how useful adult stem cells could be before advancing one or both types of research would be "irresponsible." In their prepared testimony, the ethicists Arthur Caplan and Glenn McGee note, "The fact is that no one can be sure what research on adult stem cells will produce. . . . It is absolutely true that embryonic stem cell research is also so new that it can only accurately be described as promising. . . . Adult stem cell research is neither an alternative to or substitute for embryonic stem cell research. If the goals are to repair broken, damaged or dying cells in human beings than [*sic*] both lines of research must be pursued" (*Stem Cells, 2001,* 2001, p. 103). Caplan and McGee argue that both areas of research are too new to be described as anything other than promising. Neither research area can replace the other one, and because of this, researchers and the government funding them should try to realize the promise of both. Senator Edward Kennedy reemphasizes this point in a hearing held in early September 2001: "I believe that research on adult stem cells should proceed in parallel with a vigorous research program on embryonic stem cells" (*Stem Cell Research,* 2001, p. 58).

All three equivocal responses appear in the months surrounding President Bush's decision on ES cell research, a period of intense debate about the respective value of adult and ES cell research. As noted earlier, *kairos* poses risks as well as opportunities, especially risks for speakers in the present moment who would try to create an opportunity for stem cell research. This risk is intensified after a decision has been made about ES cell research, so these equivocal responses withhold judgment on ES and adult stem cells. They do so because they lack the information necessary to make an "objective" assessment of the cells' potential. These statements allow the rhetors, who are not biologists, to attempt to contain the risk of speaking on scientific issues by creating a position that obviates a need to consider the extant scientific information or issues surrounding the two stem cell types. Instead of reasserting or refuting the claims based on the hierarchy argument from science—and related claims about self-renewal and the isolation of stem cells—the equivocal claim avoids involvement with these issues, thus removing the need to make judgments about different options for funding stem cell research from the realm of politics. Political actors who claim the equivocal position are not required to decide which strands of scientific research—those emphasizing the potency of adult stem cells or those questioning it—deserve attention: They can simply claim that research is ongoing or evolving and promise to support all relevant research.

Scientists occasionally make equivocal claims. These appear even less frequently than equivocations by nonscientific rhetors, and they occur earlier in the debate. For example, Dr. Darwin Prockop, who studies adult stem cells at Tulane University, testifies, "We simply cannot be certain in advance which therapies will work and which will not. . . . In my opinion, it would be a serious mistake to stop all research on human embryonic stem cells and tissues because of the exciting discoveries my laboratory and others have recently made about adult stem cells. We are simply not ready for a moon shot–like strategy in which we place all our bets on adult stem cells" (*Stem Cell Research, part 3,* 2000, p. 90). Prockop argues against stopping ES cell research because of research produced in his laboratory as well as in the labs of others. While it is uncertain which types of research and which therapies will be effective, choosing only adult stem cells decreases the likelihood of developing therapies. The strongest claim that can be made is that both avenues of research must be pursued in order to produce medical therapies. A different scientific use of the equivocation strategy comes from Dr. James Thomson, the biologist who first isolated human ES cells. He claims, "The debate about whether adult or embryonic stem cells is [*sic*] better is a political debate not shared by mainstream stem cell biologists" (*Stem Cells, 2001,* 2001, p. 148). His testimony attempts to demarcate science from politics: Debates about which category of stem cells is better come from politics instead of science, he argues. Thomson tries to portray science as apolitical and thus detached from messy policy debates. In both cases, the scientific rhetors try to divorce scientific practice from the policy debate in order to inoculate specific projects from the risk of political interference. Prockop tries to dissociate his work on adult stem cells from claims by opponents of ES cell research. Thomson goes further and tries to separate all scientific work from debates about ES and adult stem cells.

Equivocation intensifies the separation of specific scientific projects and the claims produced by that work from the policy debate and its scientistic idiom. This runs counter to attempts by other scientists to make the policy debate adhere to the findings of science. While this might be an attempt of scientists to have it both ways—a desire to tell the public, "Listen to what we say but do not interfere in what we do"—this form of equivocation recognizes the danger the policy debate poses to specific scientific projects. Congress has the power to eliminate projects by cutting federal funding for them and by making certain practices illegal. While unlikely, Congress could have made it illegal to derive ES cells from human embryos. Scientists might want to influence the debate, but in doing so they face the risk that their engagement endangers the scientific projects for which they advocate.

Equivocations in news discourse take two forms. First, some newspaper articles declare that the information needed to judge the relative value of various stem cells does not exist yet. *The Omaha World Herald* reports, "Researchers still don't know the full potential of either source of stem cells" (Olson, 2000d). *The Washington Post* observes, "There are big differences among stem cells from embryos, fetuses and adult tissue, and scientists don't know much about any of them" ("Cadavers Are Latest Source," 2000). Such statements recognize the hierarchy of cell types, the hierarchy's ambiguities, and the contingent nature of current knowledge about stem cells: Scientists recognize differences between stem cell types, but the nature of the cells and their differences is not fully understood. These equivocal presentations absolve readers from having to make decisions about what to believe concerning stem cell potency: The story simultaneously presents material to support the case that adult stem cells are more powerful while also presenting the case that ES cells are more powerful. Readers can fall back onto positions they might have already articulated about the value of ES cells for medical applications or objections to using embryonic human life in research. These equivocations begin rendering *any* argument based on the hierarchy moot.

Second, some articles report on the knowledge gap identified in the first strategy and then present scientists who use that gap to draw conclusions about science policy. After discussing recently published work on adult stem cells, an April 2000 *Washington Post* article notes, "Many researchers warn against cutting off embryo and fetal research before finding out which cells offer the most medical potential" (Weiss, 2000a). The article closes with an observation by researcher Fred Gage: "'My bottom line is we should not be making policy decisions about which cells are best, or which kind of research to support, because we don't have enough data to make that decision. . . . It could be a mistake to limit our inquiries to just one kind of cell'" (Weiss, 2000a). A 2002 article from *The Christian Science Monitor* also closes with similar observations from a scientist: "'If we stop in any line and focus on one, and then we find out we're wrong, think of the years of potential therapy that will have been lost'" (Spotts, 2002). Another 2002 article presents an equivocation like the one deployed by Prockop in congressional hearings of 2000. In responding to press releases from Sen. Sam Brownback (R–KS) declaring that Dr. Catherine Verfaillie's research obviated the need for ES cells, Verfaillie tells the Minneapolis *Star Tribune* that "it is too soon to say whether adult or embryo stem cells will cure any diseases," and the article later notes, "research and advocacy groups that favor federal funding of embryo research said both adult and embryonic stem cell research needs to be pursued" (Marcotty & Lerner, 2002). This type of news equivocation recognizes the limited knowledge currently available to scientists and to the public. It turns to stem cell researchers who claim the limited scope of knowledge means that current knowledge should not be the basis for policy and a broad research agenda is justified. Uncertainty creates risk for speakers who project a future filled with medical applications produced by one type of stem cell or the other. This risk is managed by calling for further research, but such a maneuver risks undermining the probity of any policy specifically based on recent research. Yet, even here, there is still a level of balanced news coverage, as scientific calls for further research into ES and adult stem cells are contrasted with demands from opponents like Sam Brownback to end ES cell research.

Conclusion

While the public depends on scientific language and argument, embodied in the scientistic idiom, it minimizes its dependence on specific scientific claims. Arguments based on a hierarchy of stem cell types embody this tension between borrowing the general form and the specific content of science. In the debate over ES cell research that took place from 1998 through early 2002, the mechanics of potency were unclear. Scientific uses of "potency" and prefixes to denote levels of power were not substantially different from etymological definitions or commonplace understandings of the terms.

Scientific use of hierarchy depends on commonplace understandings of the terms to organize the various types of cells discovered. Positing the relationship between cell types as one of potency transforms the differences between stem cell types into differences of degree rather than differences of kind. A continuous hierarchy of potency establishes that all stem cells are similar in their most fundamental capacity to become multiple cell types. This provides scientists a common framework to discuss findings generated by experiments with different cell types. Based on these definitions, scientific rhetors can develop claims and arguments about the various cells. Scientists can use the overall hierarchy and the implied similarity of all stem cell types to unify disparate research projects and develop an overarching set of concepts and research questions to drive future research: Questions about the nature of potency and how it diminishes and increases with various cell types come to the fore. The potency hierarchy also allows proponents and opponents to argue that different cell types meet the various needs the scientists and the public want stem cells to fulfill. Proponents of ES cell research develop their arguments from a simple reading of the hierarchy. Since ES cells are defined as having greater potency than adult stem cells, and since potency represents the quality necessary for performing research, developing drug screens, and creating medical applications, then ES cells are the best option for continued research and for receiving federal funding. While opponents of ES cell research could also perform a simple reading and argue that adult stem cells have enough potency, that they are good enough to meet our needs, they usually perform a more complex rhetorical operation.

The hierarchy and its specific names for various power levels (pluripotency, multipotency, and so on) generate ambiguity. The overlap between the meanings of the prefixes "pluri-" and "multi-" is considerable. This ambiguity is no mere misunderstanding of science by nonscientists: From 1998 until 2004, there was considerable ambiguity about the nature of potency, especially pluripotency, and the mechanisms that made stem cell potency possible. Scientists, as well as politicians and journalists, turn this ambiguity into a resource for rhetorical invention by using the ambiguities to generate claims about the plasticity and potency of adult stem cells and new super-powerful classes of progenitor cells (which were placed on the hierarchy at an initially low level). These arguments amplify the assumptions of the hierarchy. Scientific uses of ambiguity amplify the assumption that all stem cell types are fundamentally similar, and repeated use of claims grounded in the overlap and ambiguities of the hierarchy generate further hypotheses for research. Taking their cue from this research and the inherent ambiguities in the hierarchy, opponents can argue that adult stem cells have the *same* potency as ES cells, making them a viable and an ethically uncontentious route to achieving medical applications and cures for disease.

It is in response to uses of the hierarchy and its ambiguities that scientists and nonscientists try to modify the "distance" between the scientistic idiom and the science of stem cell research. Faced with arguments for adult stem cells based in a fundamental ambiguity about adult stem cell potency, some scientists use their authority as scientists to claim that ES cells are the better route to medical therapies, while others deploy fragments of discourse from the scientific literature. Here, scientists try to make the public debate hew closely to the scientific discourse. When nonscientists respond to ambiguity, they return to the *kairos* of application and worry that focusing on adult stem cells will be a fruitless search, but these arguments also depend on scientific authority to make their claims stronger. Yet, scientists will also make equivocal arguments that try to establish a firm boundary between science and public policy. This occurs because of the uncertainty around the ultimate policy outcome and the emotionally charged nature of some discourse in this debate. Scientists who use a strategy of equivocation try to protect scientific projects from political interference. Politicians use equivocation as a covering strategy that allows all potential research avenues to be funded: It allows politicians to take credit for any research that leads to successful therapies.

Yet, equivocation has limits. First, it works to persuade only audiences that do not treat the personhood of early-stage embryos as an absolute. If an audience were convinced by abortion-inspired arguments about ES cells, then equivocation would not work. Yet the American public had (and still has) a wide range of attitudes toward abortion and ES cells, and the equivocal argument likely has some traction. Second, equivocation assumes that funding is constant and maintained at the rate of inflation each year: If funding is limited, it might not be possible to cover multiple avenues of research. While the strategy of equivocation keeps research avenues open and comports with the attitudes of a majority of Americans, Congress never enacts any policy regarding stem cell research. This is left to the executive branch, and President Bush's decision on August 9, 2001.

6

Stalemate and the Idioms of Science-Based Controversy

George W. Bush's Manichean Idiom and
Barack Obama's Return to a Scientistic Idiom

On August 9, 2001, President George W. Bush delivered his first televised policy address to the nation. He announced his policy for ES cell research, what the administration called a compromise policy that allowed funding for research *only* on ES cells that had been derived prior to his speech. The incessant drumbeat of criticism from both opponents and proponents of ES cell research began immediately after the speech aired. While compromises will always leave both sides somewhat dissatisfied with the outcome, this speech and the policy it announces are particularly problematic for two reasons. First, the speech is untimely—it fails to have an appropriate *kairos,* the proper time and opening to effectively persuade. Second, the speech veered away from the scientistic idiom used in other forums, and it presented the debate in a Manichean idiom that undercut the possibility of finding the grounds for compromise.

President Bush's speech on ES cell research exacerbated the divide between opponents and proponents by presenting both sides of the debate as inexorably joined to religion or science and by not managing to adjudicate the claims of both sides to create the space for successful compromise. The policy his speech announced produced a stalemate: Public debate repeated the arguments by definition established prior to Bush's speech and maintained a strong science-versus-religion divide, while scientific research performed an argument about definition aimed at clarifying and reifying the concepts extant in the research and also worked to produce ES cells that circumvented the restrictions of the Bush policy. This state of affairs continued until March 3, 2009, when President Barack Obama established a new policy on ES cell research that he articulated in a scientistic idiom.

The Early Presidency of George W. Bush

Many have noted that George W. Bush's tenure in the White House is a tale of two presidencies. The first is a pre-9/11 presidency in which the president took office having lost the popular vote by a slim margin, lacking the mandate to push forward many of his programs, and facing a Senate controlled by the Democrats. The second is the post-9/11 presidency during which, as a wartime president, Bush wielded extraordinary political power. Commentators have enumerated the various challenges Bush's pre-9/11 presidency faced (Frum, 2003; Hilliard, Lansford, & Watson, 2004; Hult & Walcott, 2007; Kraus, McMahon, & Rankin, 2004). One issue is especially pertinent for understanding the process that led to Bush's August 2001 speech on stem cell research: perceptions of his intellectual ability. According to Campbell (2004), "In the 2000 election, George W. Bush had been portrayed as not intellectually up to the presidency" (p. 21). Hult and Walcott (2007) note that Bush was "seen widely as an intellectual lightweight" (p. 364), and Kirtley (2004) discusses speculation that Bush is dyslexic. Bush and his staff had to alter this perception and reassure Americans that the president was capable of addressing the complex issues the nation would face.

Bush and his staff chose the issue of ES cell research, believing it would be an ideal topic in which the president could show he was intellectually capable of addressing complex issues and engaging policy debates. To have the president successfully address such a multifaceted issue involving entrenched political constituencies, intense ethical debate, and complex, innovative science would eliminate doubts about his intellect. During the month leading up to his decision, White House staff emphasized the president's direct engagement with the most complex aspects of the ES cell debate. In June, White House chief of staff Andrew Card discussed the president's deliberations about stem cell research with reporters: "He's actually put quite a bit of time into this. . . . He's talked with ethicists. He's talked with scientists, doctors. He is spending a lot of time. It should not be treated as an easy issue" (Gilbert & Skiba, 2001). In mid-July, CNN reported, "Senior White House aides have tried to project an image of a studious President, one who is taking opinions from all sides, one who met just last night with a group of bioethicists" ("D.C. Police Search," 2001). In the hours leading up to Bush's speech, NBC News told audiences, "For months, the president has agonized over a choice that has tremendous political consequences. Sources say he's even raised the dilemma during unrelated meetings" ("President Bush to Announce," 2001). The day after, they reported, "Top advisors were eager to portray this compromise announcement as the result of a thoughtful and deeply engaged leader" ("Political Reaction," 2001).

While the complexity of the issue made ES cell research an ideal case for debunking negative images of the president's intellect, other facets of the issue made it less than ideal. First, during the 2000 presidential campaign, Bush had opposed funding for ES cell research. This was especially clear after President Bill Clinton announced a policy in August allowing the NIH to fund ES cell research as long as those funds did not pay for the derivation of ES cells from embryos ("Controversy Surrounding," 2001; "Embryos Created," 2001; "Federal

Guidelines," 2000; Leonard, 2000). Then, President Bush reiterated his opposition to federal funding in a May 18, 2001, letter to the Culture of Life Foundation, an anti-abortion group ("Controversy Surrounding," 2001; "President Bush Says," 2001).

Second, Bush takes a long time to reach a decision. Immediately after taking office, Bush put the implementation of Clinton's ES cell research policy on hold, pending a review of its legal basis (Stolberg, 2001c). In March, the administration announced it would make a decision within a week (Goldstein & Allen, 2001). A similar announcement was made in late June ("Michelle Kiley Discusses," 2001). In July, the decision was repeatedly described as being a few weeks away ("Controversy Surrounding," 2001; "Influential Senator Bill Frist," 2001; "President Bush's Appeal," 2001), and it was finally made in early August. The long delay between suspending the Clinton administration rules and producing a new policy could make the Bush administration appear indecisive instead of deliberative and thoughtful, and the seven months of intense debate led to a public fairly polarized by this issue.

Third, the debate about ES cell research creates a split in the Republican Party. Anti-abortion groups, the Roman Catholic Church, and Republican members of the House of Representatives like Dick Armey (R-TX), Tom DeLay (R-TX), and J. C. Watts (R-OK) opposed federal funding for ES cell research, but Republicans like Nancy Reagan and Arlen Specter as well as anti-abortion foes like Orrin Hatch and Bill Frist generally supported ES cell research, with some limits on the derivation of ES cells from embryos and a ban on therapeutic cloning. In fact, at a July 18 Senate hearing, Frist presented his own potential policy for ES cell research that allowed the NIH to fund research using any ES cell line available, as long as those cell lines were produced *only* from embryos destined to be discarded (*Stem Cells, 2001,* 2001, pp. 17–18). Against the backdrop of these challenges, President Bush gave a speech on August 9 in which he tried to traverse the conflicting opinions about this research in the nation and within his own party.

Defining the Middle Ground out of Existence

In his speech on August 9, 2001, President Bush portrays the serious moral and social issues at play in ES cell research and tries to perform the careful deliberation his spokespeople have claimed occurred over the previous seven months. In defining what ES cells are and the issues surrounding them, he borrows opposing definitional fragments from opponents and proponents of the debate and recasts them as religious and scientific claims, thus defining the middle ground of compromise he desperately seeks out of existence.

Bush begins the speech by thanking his audience for their attention as he addresses "a complex and difficult issue, an issue that is one of the most profound of our time" (Bush, 2001, para. 1).[1] He notes that ES cells could save lives, but that some people have objections to that research because it destroys embryos: "At its core, this issue forces us to confront fundamental questions about the beginnings of life and the ends of science. It lies at a difficult moral intersection, juxtaposing the need to protect life in all its phases with the prospect of saving and improving life in all its stages" (para. 16). These issues highlight the "great promise and great peril" of ES cell research (para. 23), and this mix of danger and opportunity justifies his repeated assertion that this decision was made with "great care" (para. 23, 29).

Bush also highlights the broad reach of this issue. Discussion of the issues surrounding ES cell research is not limited to laboratories: "It is agonized over by parents and many couples as they try to have children, or to save children already born. The issue is debated within the church, with people of different faiths, even many of the same faith coming to different conclusions. Many people are finding that the more they know about stem cell research, the less certain they are about the right ethical and moral conclusions" (para. 2–3). People from all walks of life confront and are confused by this issue, Bush claims. This division and debate are also reflected in the president's "deeply held beliefs" that shaped his position (para. 21): He is "a strong supporter of science and technology" (para. 21), who also believes "human life is a sacred gift from our Creator" (para. 22).

Bush's repeated depiction of intellectual and moral division sets the stage for a speech structured as a two-sided argument between moral and scientific concerns. In considering the major issues raised by proponents and opponents, a Solomon-like Bush will make the proper cut. In developing this two-sided argument, Bush turns to the extant debate in the scientific, scholarly, and public arenas, but he deploys the definitional fragments and strategies in a way that recasts arguments originally presented in a scientistic idiom as either scientific or religious, thus leaving no middle ground available for compromise.

First, Bush defines ES cells by their potential ends when he discusses the medical applications ES cells might produce. Near the beginning of the speech, he notes, "Based on preliminary work that has been privately funded, scientists believe further research using stem cells offers great promise that could help improve the lives of those who suffer from many terrible diseases—from juvenile diabetes to Alzheimer's, from Parkinson's to spinal cord injuries" (para. 6). Later, he remarks, "Research offers hope that millions of our loved ones may be cured of a disease and rid of their suffering. I have friends whose children suffer from juvenile diabetes. Nancy Reagan has written me about President Reagan's struggle with Alzheimer's. My own family has confronted the tragedy of childhood leukemia. And, like all Americans, I have great hope for cures" (para. 21). Bush highlights the hope scientists have of producing medical applications from

ES cells and how that research offers that same hope to all Americans. He refers to some of the diseases most often mentioned as targets for stem cell therapy—Alzheimer's disease, juvenile diabetes, Parkinson's disease, and spinal cord injury. Yet, his use of the terms "preliminary," "believe," "promise," and "hope" throughout these passages highlights the ambivalence in this appeal. The use of "preliminary" and "believe" in the first passage emphasizes the possibility that ES cell research will never realize the promise of medical applications, and this potential for failure is clearly highlighted later in the speech when he says, "No one can be certain that the science will live up to the hope it has generated" (para. 22). After he warns about the possibility of false hope, the next paragraph provides the example of fetal tissue research as a scientific endeavor that did not live up to its initial promise, and he uses that example to justify proceeding with "great care" (para. 23). The appeal to medical applications—the use of *kairos* to define ES cells by a possible future end—opens up the twin possibilities of success and failure. Bush highlights both of these possibilities without distinguishing between them. While it allows him to justify a cautious policy, "great care" does not specify the exact nature of the cautious approach to be taken, or how "care" justifies Bush's policy rather than Clinton's policy or proposals like those from Senator Frist.

The lack of distinction or discrimination between the two sides of the argument continues with his presentation of definitions of the embryo. Bush identifies the issues he believes are at the heart of the ES cell debate. In elaborating on the nature of those issues, he presents the dissociation of blastocysts from other stages of human life, and then offers the opponent's definition, based on an *incrementum* placing all human life on the same continuum:

> On the first issue, are these embryos human life—well, one researcher told me he believes this five-day-old cluster of cells is not an embryo, not yet an individual, but a pre-embryo. He argued that it has the potential for life, but it is not a life because it cannot develop on its own.
>
> An ethicist dismissed that as a callous attempt at rationalization. Make no mistake, he told me, that cluster of cells is the same way you and I, and all the rest of us, started our lives. One goes with a heavy heart if we use these, he said, because we are dealing with the seeds of the next generation. (para. 13–14)

Following these two paragraphs, Bush raises the issue of "spare embryos":

> And to the other crucial question, if these are going to be destroyed anyway, why not use them for good purpose. . . . Many argue these embryos

are byproducts of a process that helps create life, and we should allow couples to donate them to science so they can be used for good purpose instead of wasting their potential. Others will argue there's no such thing as excess life, and the fact that a living being is going to die does not justify experimenting on it or exploiting it as a natural resource. (para. 15)

While Bush's presentation here reiterates claims about the status of the "embryo" and "spare embryos" already in public circulation, he recasts those definitions, *all* of which appeared in a scientistic idiom as either scientific or moral: A scientist offers a claim that a blastocyst is not an embryo, while an ethicist counters that definition, and the situation becomes murkier with the issue of spare embryos which has "many" saying one thing while "others" offer a rebuttal. Additionally, the placement of the two positions in this argument is ambiguous: If one knew nothing about the president's stance on embryonic life from the abortion debate, then they could equally argue that the first position presented (that of the proponents) is favored or that the latter position (that of the opponents) is the stronger. Even knowing that Bush favors the pro-life position, the tension between preserving the life of the embryo and promoting research that could improve the quality of life for many people remains unresolved in this speech. Ultimately Bush decides to allow research using extant ES cell lines because "the life and death decision has already been made" (para. 24), but this decision does not explain why it is acceptable to use these embryos—these former "seeds of the next generation"—as a resource.

Bush's speech reflects the debate about stem cells that occurred in scientific and congressional discourse, but, as Kenneth Burke might note, the speech also "perfects" the debate by taking the conflicting sides to the point of stalemate (Burke, 1966). Bush deploys definitions of the embryo used by proponents and opponents: He offers claims that blastocysts are not human and that blastocysts should be regarded as human; he notes that spare embryos are considered an acceptable source for ES cells immediately before mentioning that some dismiss the idea of using spare embryos as a source for ES cells. While two-sided argumentation presents both sides of a debate, one side's definitions—and claims and in many cases of compromise, both sides' definitions and claims—are modified, allowing enough of the original to exist for advocates to accept the argument's conclusion while allowing a new position to develop. Bush does not offer any adjudication or modification of the claims presented, allowing them to stand in stark contrast to each other.

This unresolved conflict between the different definitional fragments Bush has used is intensified by problems of *kairos* and problems of idiom. Bush's speech is untimely for two reasons. First, since *kairos* involves knowing when to keep silent as much as knowing when to speak, Bush's speech fails to meet or create *kairos* in his choice to speak in the first place. Bush faced serious constraints at this time: He had lost the popular vote; he was viewed as intellectually incapable of the job; and with ES cell research, he faced a division within his own party. The combination of these three challenges made the ES cell debate a poor vehicle for showcasing Bush's intellect. Second, Bush took too long to speak. While trying to use this issue as a display of presidential prudence would have been problematic in any case, the long wait for Bush's speech gave Congress the opportunity to frame the issue and define the terms of the debate. The most problematic issue here was the existence of an *alternate* plan for ES cell research articulated by a pro-life conservative. Bill Frist had offered a plan for ES cell research that allowed the use of all spare embryos. Whether intentional or not, Frist's plan redefined spare embryos as liminal objects existing between human life and "mere" cells, and this plan would allow ES cell research to go forward under strict government oversight. Given that another pro-life conservative had offered a plan for ES cell research less than a month before his speech, Bush's own plan, with its lack of justification for limiting ES cell research to cell lines already in existence, looks inadequate by comparison.

Bush's choice of idiom also exacerbates this problem. Bush breaks with the scientistic idiom used in congressional hearings about ES cell research and uses a Manichean idiom to present the definitions used as scientific *or* religious, which is a prevalent treatment within journalistic discourse about ES cells. Bush presents pro–ES cell definitions as ones produced by scientists or as being related to scientific pursuits, while anti–ES cell definitions are defined as ethical and religious. Presenting the two sides in this way furthers the conceptual distance between them. There is no clear connection between religious and scientific standards for judgment and no way to bring the two into coherent conversation. By eschewing the scientistic idiom, Bush sets aside a mode of public deliberation that allows for linking real definitions with ideological commitments, and he increases the difficulty of crafting a coherent compromise.

Bush presents both sides of the debate about ES cell research in order to establish that he is thoughtful and engaged in policy debates, but to create that perception successfully, the resulting policy must be thoughtful and coherent. While viable compromise options did exist, Bush's policy is not one of them. Nonetheless, Bush had the power to institute this policy, and in doing so, he generated further debate and discourse about ES cell research.

Shifting and Expanding the Debate

George W. Bush announced his policy on ES cell research during his first televised address to the nation. While the grounds for that policy were undermined by his inability to resolve the tension between the conflicting definitions he presented, the speech did generate further discourse. Some of it returned to the same definitional grounds that had occupied previous congressional and media discourse, but an even greater portion of the discourse focused on new issues, such as the validity of the August 9, 2001, deadline for funding, the number and viability of stem cell lines, and concerns that patents on ES cell technology would lead to a monopoly on research. Bush's speech shifted public debate from arguments about definition to a focus on the details of procedure and policy.

Immediate Reaction

In the immediate aftermath of Bush's speech, administration spokespeople emphasized the president's role in designing this policy and their perception of the policy as a compromise. Opponents and proponents of ES cell research criticized the policy, but the type and intensity of the objections from both camps differed wildly, with proponents decrying the decision as driven by politics and incapable of promoting ES cell research and opponents reiterating their moral objections to the research.

After Bush presented his policy, aides portrayed the decision as a compromise on a tough issue, a compromise in whose creation the president played a central role. The day after his decision, CNN reported, "White House aides say President Bush is very comfortable with his decision, which effectively positions him in the middle ground of this debate" ("Bush's Stem Cell Decision," 2001). CBS's John Roberts said, "President Bush's decision last night was an attempt to place himself in the political center in the debate over embryonic stem cell research" ("Debate over President Bush's," 2001). News reports highlight the efforts of the administration to present the decision as a compromise. The language of compromise implies Bush is engaged with the issues, which some reports repeat in other language. The language of compromise also allows the administration to dismiss some of the immediate objections to the policy: During a press conference, Karen Hughes stated, "One of the things you learn as President is that you are not able to make all people happy all the time" ("Bush Defends Decision," 2001).

In trying to dismiss or minimize the impact of criticism, the administration was responding to a variety of criticisms. Journalists were reporting proponents' objections that the decision was political posturing and bad policy. According to House minority leader Richard Gephardt (D-MO), "Once again, the president has done the bare minimum in order to try and publicly posture himself with the majority of the Americans . . . but Americans know this is not the decision that the science community needs to go forward full force" (Goldstein & Allen, 2001). CBS's Elizabeth Kaledin reported, "Many doctors . . . see the President's plan as nothing more than a quick political fix that won't really help the science evolve" ("People Who Are," 2001). *The New York Times* reported, "For months, scientists have hoped President Bush would set an important precedent by allowing federal financing for embryonic stem cell research. Mr. Bush did just that tonight, but leading experts were sorely disappointed by his decision, describing it as a baby step, rather than a giant leap, for medical research" (Stolberg, 2001b). The immediate responses of proponents cast Bush's decision as "political" and therefore more interested in appealing to popular opinion instead of providing the necessary policies to realize the promise of ES cell research.

Opponents of ES cell research were harsher in their criticism. In an interview with CNN, the Family Research Council's Ken Connor declared, "We believe that it flies in the face of his promise not to engage in research that involves the destruction of live embryonic human beings" ("Bush Defends Decision," 2001). House majority whip Tom DeLay (R-TX) warned, "This initial research may ultimately serve as a pretext for vastly expanded research that does require the destruction of new living embryos" (Goldstein & Allen, 2001). The United States Conference of Catholic Bishops called the decision "morally unacceptable" (Page & Hall, 2001), and in a press conference, Bay Buchanan, sister of former presidential candidate Pat Buchanan, claimed that Bush "would have been a far greater leader, a far greater spokesperson, a far greater voice for the unborn had he shut that door entirely" ("Debate over President Bush's Stem Cell Research Funding Decision," 2001).

Opponents presenting their arguments in the media use moral language to condemn Bush's policy. Proponents have access to equally powerful arguments to call for an expansion of research, but their responses appear moderate. While the policy restricts the lines that can be used for research, it does allow the research to go forward. Bush has modified the position he articulated as a candidate enough to allow some research to continue, and he has given researchers access to previously unavailable funding for some projects. Although this partial victory led to an initially moderate response by proponents and the intense objections of opponents, the proponents will ultimately intensify their arguments as they consider the ramifications of the Bush policy. Among the concerns addressed, the two most prominent are the number of stem cell lines available and the impact of patents on this research area.

Stem Cell Lines

As people addressed the implications of the Bush policy, they began to produce more discourse about stem cells that moved beyond argument *from, about,* or *by* definition. While many of these concerns were raised as objections to the Bush policy (for example, "The policy won't work or was falsely sold to the American people because of X, Y, and Z"), the use and circulation of these fragments produces pedagogical, as well as policy-related, discourse. The discourse concerning stem cell "lines" highlights the pedagogical circulation of these new fragments as well as their use in objections to the Bush policy.

In his speech, Bush claimed that "60 genetically diverse stem cell lines" existed (para. 24). Bush's speech and the NIH report *Stem Cells* (National Institutes of Health, 2001) both use the phrase "stem cell lines," but they do not provide a specific definition of the term. Television news reports detailing Bush's policy and the immediate reaction of proponents of the research refer to stem cell lines but do not provide a description (see, for example, "Debate over President Bush's Stem Cell Research Funding Decision," 2001; "National Institutes of Health Claims," 2001; "President Bush Interviewed," 2001; "President Bush to Announce," 2001). Initial newspaper coverage, perhaps because the medium allows more time to discuss issues and is not in direct competition with television news to report breaking news first, takes time to describe stem cell lines. *USA Today* notes, "A single stem-cell line represents a colony of continually dividing cells derived from a single early-stage embryo. To create a stem-cell line, an embryo must be destroyed. But existing stem cell lines can produce an indefinite supply of cells" (Friend, 2001d). A few days later, another *USA Today* article describes stem cell lines as "clusters of cells that descended from a single embryo" (Manning, 2001). The language of stem cell "colonies" is most frequently used by newspapers (Ackerman & Roth, 2001; Brown, 2001; Connolly, Gillis, & Weiss, 2001; Friend, 2001f; Seelye, 2001; Stolberg, 2001b; Vergano, 2001b). Commonsense understandings of colonies drawn from history and politics, as well as biology (for instance, a colony of honeybees), thus begin to shape the reader's perception of stem cell lines.

These pedagogical moments are a component of challenges to the viability of Bush's stem cell policy. First, some questioned whether Bush's claim that 60 stem cell lines existed was in fact accurate. In the days following Bush's speech, news media reported that scientists and proponents of ES cell research were surprised by Bush's statement. ABC's Jackie Judd reported, "Many scientists we talked to today seemed surprised, even a little baffled, by the President's claim that there are 60 stem cell lines" ("National Institutes of Health Claims," 2001). As the month progressed, the concern about the number of existing stem cell lines became exaggerated: "To limit researchers to 60 cell lines, critics say, is like telling mathematicians they can pursue their studies but they can never use numbers bigger than 10" (Connolly et al., 2001).

On August 25, the NIH announced the locations of all 60 stem cell lines to which Bush had referred in his speech ("Embryonic Stem Cell Research,"

2001; Friend, 2001c; "Health Officials Pinpoint," 2001; "NIH Takes a Look," 2001), but concerns about the number and availability of lines continued. *USA Today* noted, "Some researchers suggested the number is inflated because some of the lines are of too poor quality to use fully or are tied up in legal claims" (Friend, 2001c). This problem was exacerbated when Health and Human Services (HHS) secretary Tommy Thompson announced that only 24 of the 60 lines Bush had referenced were available for research (*Stem Cell Research,* 2001; see also "Congress Debates," 2001; "Less Stem Research" 2001; Lore, 2001). Concerns were raised in Senate hearings on Bush's policy (*Stem Cell Research,* 2001; *Cloning, 2001,* 2001). In a December 2001 hearing, Senator Specter declared, "My own view is that the limiting of the federal funding on stem cell research to the approximately 70 lines in existence as of August 9 is tying the hands of scientists" (*Cloning, 2001,* 2001, p. 3). Dr. Bert Vogelstein argued in the same hearing that "research to produce new stem cell lines would be needed to take this area from strictly a research arena to a clinical arena" (*Cloning, 2001,* 2001, p. 39). Proponents of ES cell research were concerned from the beginning that the number of stem cell lines Bush claimed existed was incorrect and that, even if the number was accurate, more cell lines would be needed to realize the promise of medical applications.

A second concern focuses on the quality of the extant stem cell lines. During an interview with ABC News, Dr. John Gearhart explained, "We don't know the source. We don't know what the criteria were to say that they are, in fact, stem cell lines. We just know nothing about them" ("President Bush Interviewed," 2001). A *Washington Post* article highlights the importance of the number and quality of stem cell lines: "The number and variety of cell lines available is important because stem cells are highly finicky and quite volatile. Cell lines can 'crash'—or die—at any moment, or they can spontaneously turn into specialized cells, rendering them useless for later work" (Connolly et al., 2001). This issue was raised again with the NIH announcement of the location of the 60 stem cell lines. The following exchange occurred during an ABC News report on the NIH announcement:

CHARLES GIBSON: Do the scientists agree that all 60 of these lines are real and usable for research?

JOHN COCHRAN: They're not sure that all 60 are usable. ("NIH Takes a Look," 2001)

This concern is also echoed in congressional discourse on the issue. During the first hearing following Bush's decision, Senator Specter observed, "We know very little about the quality of those existing stem cell lines, except that leading scientists state that up to one-third of them may be so fragile that they will be of no use to any researcher" (*Stem Cell Research,* 2001).[2]

By limiting federal funding for ES cell research to 60 stem cell lines derived before he gave his speech, Bush generated a discursive fragment that would be mobilized and circulated in discourse about, and discourse critical of, his decision. The issue of stem cell lines challenges the viability of Bush's policy on two fronts: whether the lines he mentioned actually exist and represent a sufficient number for viable research and whether the quality of the stem cell lines will make them viable for research.

Patents

In addition to the number of cell lines allowed under the Bush policy, the ownership of those lines becomes an issue proponents raise to challenge the viability of Bush's plan. Two days after Bush announced his policy, ABC's Bob Woodruff reported, "Another concern to US scientists is that private corporations now own many of the existing stem cell supplies. So in the US, the few companies that own those cell lines can exert tremendous control over federally-funded research" ("Limited Stem Cell Research," 2001). Ten days later, a *Boston Globe* article claims, "The ownership of many of the lines are [*sic*] shrouded in secrecy" (Mishra, 2001). After the NIH identifies the locations of the 60 stem cell lines, a CBS news story explains why patents and ownership are important issues: "The concern is that the list, in effect, grants monopoly rights to private companies, who will benefit from federally-funded discoveries" ("Health Officials Pinpoint," 2001). The implications of patents on ES cells are addressed at greatest length in an August 18 ABC News report. Weekend news anchor Cynthia McFadden opens the piece: "There is more controversy this weekend over the president's decision on stem cell research. At the center of the debate, the power of patents. Virtually all scientific discoveries from drugs to medical devices are patented by their inventors, including human embryonic stem cells" ("Stem Cell Research and Patents," 2001). After describing how the University of Wisconsin has patents on ES cells and the techniques used to derive them and how Geron, a California-based biotechnology company, funded the research, reporter Deborah Amos notes, "Scientists are already working on the approved stem cells. They are free to research, and publish anything they find. But if one of them discovers a cure for, say, Parkinson's disease, and then wants to market the breakthrough, Geron and the University of Wisconsin have a say over who profits. . . . The White House says the president was fully briefed on the patent issue. And he understood the implications for the decision he was making" ("Stem Cell Research and Patents," 2001). This news story uses its brief primer on patents and contemporary scientific research to flesh out concerns about how patents give certain organizations power over the course of stem cell research: The patent and the attendant licensing rights allow Geron and the University of Wisconsin to determine how discoveries are marketed and who can profit from them, and these considerations, which the president knew, can negatively impact scientists' willingness to engage in this research (see also Vergano, 2001a).

The issue of patents and intellectual property is raised during the first hearing on stem cell research after Bush's speech. There, Senator Specter observes, "We are just beginning to learn which researchers and companies throughout the world have ownership of existing stem cell lines, but we have little knowledge of their property rights, their willingness to share or license the use of those lines to other researchers, or whether the donors of those embryos have given the requisite informed consent" (*Stem Cell Research,* 2001).[3] Harvard's Dr. Douglas Melton also discusses the impact of patents and private corporate ownership of many stem cell lines:

> A separate issue concerns whether the cell lines will be made available to federally funded researchers in a timely manner and without restrictions on their use for research. It is noteworthy that most of the entities that have isolated the sixty+ human embryonic stem cell lines are companies with proprietary and commercial interests. In addition, there are relevant patents on some of the cells that may further restrict their distribution and use. (*Stem Cell Research,* 2001, p. 63)

While Bush's speech did not address the issue of patents, it comes to the fore because Bush has limited the number of stem cell lines that qualify for federal funding. If the work on these cells leads to medical applications, the owners of those stem cell lines will have the ability to limit or control how they are developed and made available to the public.

Defending Bush Policy

As proponents for ES cell research are attacking the Bush decision on several fronts, the Bush administration tries to manage the resistance to the policy. The majority of the defense is global in nature, defending the overall policy as the best choice available. This defense begins the day after Bush announces his policy and is led by Bush himself in an interview with ABC's Claire Shipman:

SHIPMAN: Some people are saying that compromise, in this case, might not have been such a great thing because it's the worst of all worlds.

BUSH: Claire, Claire, all I can tell you is that I made the decision I thought was the right decision. I'm very comfortable with the decision, in terms of the moral line you just described, the life and death decision has already been made. ("President Bush Interviewed," 2001)

Bush emphasizes the morality of his decision, and he rearticulates his belief in that "rightness" when he threatens to veto any legislation altering his policy: "The statement I laid out is what I'm—what I—what I think is right for America, and any piece of legislation that undermines what I think is right will be vetoed" ("Bush Talks about Stem Cell Research," 2001; see also "Most Americans Satisfied," 2001). The administration also argues that advances in stem cell research and potential problems with the approved stem cells will not lead to any policy change ("Complication in President Bush's Policy," 2001; "Supporters of Both Sides Debate," 2001).

Other defenders of the Bush policy try to redefine the ends of stem cell research, the possibility of applications, by downplaying the expediency with which the research will produce cures: If the "promise" of the quickly produced cures is not feasible—if a great deal of research and caution is needed—a policy that moves slowly becomes the best course of action. This rhetorical strategy primarily appears in the September 5, 2001, hearing on Bush's policy held by the Senate Committee on Health, Education, Labor and Pensions. Senator Frist downplays the expediency of ES cell research in his testimony: "We must recognize that the field of embryonic stem cell research is young, it is early, it is pioneering; it is not yet tested. The benefits of this research, although we all attach huge hope to this particular field, have not yet been realized, and they are just possibilities" (*Stem Cell Research,* 2001, p. 7). Frist's comments reorganize the discursive fragments originally used to highlight the promise of ES cell applications. Initially, proponents of ES cell research praised it for being a new and pioneering field. Now, Frist uses those qualities to diminish claims about the expediency with which medical applications will be realized. He valorizes the promise of embryonic stem cell research, but he also emphasizes the uncertainty surrounding it. In his prepared testimony, HHS secretary Tommy Thompson also redefines ES cells to minimize the expediency attached to them. Thompson begins with the observation "we all have every right to feel hopeful about what scientists may be able to accomplish," but he closes with a cautionary note: "We have much to learn about these cells—much basic research that needs to be conducted. Clinical applications, which could possibly emerge only after considerable basic research, are years away. What is important now is that we begin the process of gaining a thorough and scientifically based understanding of the promise and potential of embryonic stem cell research" (*Stem Cell Research,* 2001, p. 23). While recognizing the advantages embryonic stem cells offer to scientists hoping to cure degenerative diseases like Parkinson's disease and diabetes, Thompson argues that "considerable" amounts of time and effort must be devoted to basic research before medical applications will be possible. Thompson minimizes the expediency of embryonic stem cell research; in contrast to the claims that medical applications will be available in a few years, Thompson implies that much work will need to be done. Since the ES cell research is not as expedient as believed, a more restricted, less urgent approach to funding and studying embryonic stem cells appears, as Thompson describes it, "wise." Despite minimizing the expediency of this research, Thompson goes on to provide a timeframe of five to eight years before medical applications could appear, the same timeframe used by proponents of embryonic stem cell research. Stem cells are defined as a means to an end. Defenders of Bush's policy redefine stem cells vis-à-vis the end of medical applications, making them a less expedient means to achieve it.

Based on this redefinition, Bush's defenders accuse proponents of overselling the promise of ES cell research. Frist warns the committee that people must be careful "not to oversell the promise of this research to the American people" (*Stem Cell Research,* 2001, p. 7). In his opening statement, Thompson argues,

> Some people want to make the grand leap from the onset of federally-funded research to the cures for Parkinson's, Alzheimer's and other diseases. If only it was that easy. It is easy to make such a leap in the emotion of this debate, but it is also inaccurate and unfair to do so.
>
> The cures for these diseases are not just around the corner—I wish they were. (*Stem Cell Research,* 2001, p. 16)

Thompson even repeats the warning that cures are "not just around the corner" during the question-and-answer session following his statement (p. 40). According to Frist and Thompson, individuals highlighting the promise of embryonic stem cell research must use caution. Applications will not appear soon, and proponents must avoid letting emotion drive them to hyperbolic claims about cures for diabetes, Parkinson's disease, and other conditions.

In the months immediately following Bush's speech, proponents and opponents of the research reiterate their previous positions on ES cell research, but they also move toward a discussion of the details and implications of Bush's policy. New lines of argument about intellectual property and the number of stem cell colonies or lines available proliferate. Ultimately, none of the issues raised prior to Bush's speech were resolved by it, and none of the issues his policy raised reached a satisfying conclusion. 9/11 and the Iraq War would minimize debates about ES cell research in political and journalistic arenas until the 2004 election, when the issue returned to some prominence. During that interim, though, scientific research continued on two fronts, and the scientific definitions of ES cells were further reified by the discourse about this research through 2009.

Reifying Definitions in Science

Scientific discourse did not develop further arguments from or by definition in the aftermath of Bush's decision. While scientists had been initially pleased that ES cell research was allowed to go forward, they began to chafe at the restrictions of Bush's policy (Daley, 2004; Drazen, 2004; Schwartz, 2006). During this time, research on ES cells fell into three broad categories. First, scientists tried to identify with greater specificity what chemical and genetic properties were unique to ES cells and what material qualities constituted ES cells' key properties, pluripotency and self-renewal (Gearhart, Pashos, & Prasad, 2007; The International Stem Cell Initiative, 2007; Tokuzawa et al., 2003; Xu et al., 2005). This category of research represents a variation on argument *about* definition. Like those arguments, this research focuses on how key concepts should be defined, but while argument about definition in the public sphere is often acrimonious and heated, these research-based variations on the argument about definition acted as an extension or clarification of previous work. For example, the International Stem Cell Initiative (2007) presented the results of a comprehensive study of 59 ES cell lines that reaffirmed the use of several chemical and genetic markers as characteristic of human ES cells. An additional difference between public arguments about definition and these research-based variants is that the scientific arguments go beyond clarification of a definitional fragment and seek to reify it. The goal is to tie concepts like "ES cell" and "pluripotency" to the results of specific chemical and genetic tests. When successful, such arguments move a definition further into the realm of "fact," increasing the apparent inevitability of a definition: It creates the appearance that an object, like ES cells, could not have been defined in any other way.

Second, scientists work to fulfill the promise of ES cell research by identifying the processes that differentiate ES cells into different types of cells and tissues. Scientists during this time made progress in differentiating ES cells from mice and humans into pancreas and heart tissue (D'Amour et al., 2006; Moretti et al., 2006; Partridge, 2006). In addition to creating cells that put science further along the path of fulfilling the promise of medical applications, scientists also focused on fulfilling the promise of research applications with the creation of stem cell lines to study specific human diseases (Jordan, Guzman, & Noble, 2006; Park et al., 2008). Research by biotechnology companies working with ES cells had progressed to the point that an FDA-approved, small-scale trial of a therapy for spinal-cord injuries was initiated in 2009, although it was delayed a few months later in response to new information from studies using animals (Bloomberg News, 2009; Stein, 2009). These research projects begin with the definition of ES cells as those capable of differentiation and self-renewal, and from there, these projects try to bring the promises of medical and research applications closer to fruition.

Third, in response to the Bush policy restrictions on deriving new ES cell lines where an embryo is destroyed, scientists work to produce ES cells, or ES-like cells, that preserve the embryo and do not arouse opposition based on definitions of the embryo as human. Some researchers produce new ES cell lines, even though they are not eligible for federal funding (Cowan et al., 2004). While this form of research does not avoid the Bush policy restrictions, the researchers argue that there is a need for these cells, regardless of federal funding limits: "At present, approximately 15 human embryonic stem-cell lines are available, and they vary considerably in their usefulness for research and the extent of their characterization" (Cowan et al., 2004, p. 1353). The lines available under the Bush policy are inadequate for research, the researchers argue, thus necessitating the creation of new ES cell lines regardless of political and ethical opposition.

Equally controversial was the work on therapeutic cloning—the production of ES cells that will not be rejected by a person's immune system through the transfer of a person's genetic material. If perfected, such a research project would alter the policy debate by realizing the promise of individually tailored stem cells for medical therapies. The initial announcement that a lab in South Korea had successfully produced ES cells using therapeutic cloning stunned scientists and politicians and raised concerns about onerous legislation making cloning technology illegal ("Highly Controversial New Advances," 2004; Hwang et al., 2004; "Recent Advances in Human Cloning," 2004). Equally stunning was the announcement that the research of Hwang Woo-Suk was a fraud ("Rise and Fall," 2005; Snyder & Loring, 2006). While the initial announcement produced excitement in the news media ("Brave New World Cloning Humans," 2004; "Recent Advances in Human Cloning," 2004; "South Korean Researchers," 2004), the fabricated method produced by Hwang and colleagues was not widely used by other researchers and did not harm the overall research on ES cells, regardless of the damage done to science's reputation (Snyder & Loring, 2006).

Another set of projects produced ES, and ES-like, cells that would hopefully circumvent objections based on concerns that ES cell derivation involved the destruction of embryos. The first study entailed removing a single cell from an eight-cell blastocyst. The removed cell became an ES cell line, while the embryo was able to reach full development (Chung et al., 2006). The second study involved genetic manipulation of an embryo so that it would never be able to develop and then could be used to derive ES cells (Meissner & Jaenisch, 2006). It was believed that embryos prevented from developing would be viewed as a morally acceptable source of stem cells. Both studies used mouse embryos but claimed the results could be extended to humans. Despite the attempt to circumvent these concerns, critics and the White House were not convinced that these studies and their alteration of embryos preserved and respected life (Cook, 2006; Solter, 2005; Weiss, 2006). A final set of research studies does circumvent these concerns: Researchers in Japan and the United States identified a set of genes that could be activated in adult cells that would allow them to become pluripotent, like ES cells (Meissner, Wernig, & Jaenisch, 2007; Okita, Ichisaka, & Yamanaka, 2007; Takahashi & Yamanaka, 2006). The induced pluripotent cells would be trumpeted as a major scientific achievement and used by both sides in the public debate on stem cell research to support their policy agendas.

Repetition and Resolution in the Public Debate

While scientific discourse did not produce new definitions, it did move the project of ES cell research forward, but public debate over ES cell research did not see similar progress as public opinion and the definitions used in the debate remained stagnant. The same definitional fragments deployed before Bush's speech were repeated in the arguments by definition from 2004 through 2008, and while some discourses and debates saw the continued use of the scientistic idiom by both sides, the use of a Manichean idiom increased and exacerbated divisions between opponents and proponents of the research.

Public discourse continued to emphasize the application of ES cells to medicine and concerns about the embryos. In describing the cloning experiments from South Korea, ABC's Ned Potter observed, "What's more, one of those embryos gave them a viable cluster of stem cells, those all-purpose cells that many doctors believe may someday cure all sorts of diseases, from diabetes to arthritis to Parkinson's" ("Brave New World Cloning Humans," 2004). *The San Diego Union-Tribune*'s story on ES cell work in southern California notes, "Human embryonic stem cells turn into all the different cell types in the body, forming tissue, blood, bone and neurons" (Somers, 2006), and Sen. Gordon Smith

(R-OR) begins a 2005 hearing with the observation that ES cell research "holds the key to potentially unlocking the secrets of diseases that have mystified scientists for years, namely Alzheimer's, Parkinson's, diabetes, cardiovascular disease and more" (*Exploring the Promise,* 2005). These definitions continue to highlight the capacity of stem cells to differentiate, which means they can potentially be used to create replacement tissues for people with a variety of illnesses.

The majority of appeals to application highlighted the suffering and challenges of individuals facing incurable diseases. This occurred most often during the 2004 election. Some news stories used the examples of ordinary people suffering from diabetes or Parkinson's disease, and this trend continued in coverage of Missouri's stem cell initiative in the 2006 election ("Inside Story," 2004; Stolberg, 2006a; "US Stem Cell Research," 2004). Overall, the most prominent examples come from the 2004 election coverage and involve discussion of Ronald Reagan, who had suffered from Alzheimer's and died on June 5 of that year, and Christopher Reeve, who was paralyzed by a back injury he suffered in 1995 and who died on October 11, 2004 ("Actor and Research Advocate," 2004; "Christopher Reeve Remembered," 2004; Kraus et al., 2004; "Nancy Reagan's Battle," 2004; "What Nancy Reagan's Future Holds," 2004). These stories of individuals continue the strategy of embodying the appeal to application in specific people, a strategy that was used prior to Bush's August 9, 2001, speech. The political power of these stories increases given the prominence of Reagan and Reeve.

Definitions focused on the embryo also appear throughout the debate. Some definitions of ES cells as harm to embryos employ the scientistic idiom. A television news story on the South Korean cloning claims features the National Right to Life committee's Douglas Johnson. He remarks, "We really see this as another giant leap toward human embryo farms in which *members of the human species* will be created in large numbers to be harvested for their parts" ("Highly Controversial New Advances," 2004; emphasis mine).[4] In opening a House Committee on Government Reform hearing, Rep. Mark Souder claims, "Embryonic stem cell research requires the destruction of living human embryos to harvest their stem cells" (*Human Cloning and Embryonic Stem Cell Research,* 2006). Later in the hearing, Dr. Richard Chole from the Washington University School of Medicine observes, "One of the central questions that our society must answer in the stem cell debate is the question of when life begins. Biologically, there has never been a question as to when human life begins. A unique human being begins at the point where the chromosomes from the egg and sperm unite to form the earliest stage of human life, the zygote. One only has to look in a textbook of human embryology to understand this fact" (*Human Cloning and Embryonic Stem Cell Research,* 2006). Each of these claims uses a scientistic idiom to define embryos as developing human life that deserves protection and ES cell research as the harm of that life. Both Johnson and Souder use the language of "harvesting" and "destruction" that featured prominently in a 2001 hearing also chaired by Souder. Johnson again borrows explicitly from science with his description of embryos as members of the human species, like others did in 2000 and 2001, and Chole turns to the authority of scientific textbooks to establish that embryos are people, just as Richard Doerflinger did in 1999.

While use of the scientistic idiom persists, the number of claims using explicitly moral language increases. A 2004 CBS News report showed President Bush on the campaign trail arguing, "Life is a creation of God, not a commodity to be exploited by man" ("US Stem Cell Research," 2004). A month later, CBS's Elizabeth Kaledin notes, "Many believe embryos are human life and consider their use in research immoral" ("Where the Presidential Candidates," 2004). During the 2006 House hearing on cloning and stem cell research, Catholic spokesperson Richard Doerflinger blurs scientistic claims into an attack on cloning and ES cell research grounded in morality. His testimony offers three lessons drawn from the South Korea cloning fraud. "The third and most important lesson is moral," he claims (*Human Cloning and Embryonic Stem Cell Research,* 2006). He argues that scientific arguments for ES cell research are based on "a utilitarian calculus that relativizes and demeans human life and other values whenever they may get in the way of the research prize." According to Doerflinger, this utilitarian calculus is unethical, and those who use it will even ignore scientific fact when it runs counter to their desires: "Government advisory panels have been forced by the evidence to concede that the early human embryo is a 'human life,' because the evidence from embryology has only become more and more persuasive on that point. They even concede that this life deserves our 'respect.' Instead of concluding that experimental destruction of this life is off limits, however, they have used a cost-benefit analysis to argue that this respect is overridden by the health needs of born persons with devastating diseases" (*Human Cloning and Embryonic Stem Cell Research,* 2006). Doerflinger argues that given this willingness to ignore scientific and moral certitudes that would otherwise force people to recognize the rights of unborn human persons, no moral principle is safe: "We should not be surprised when an ethic that dismisses 'Thou shalt not kill' in the quest for cures applies the same calculus to 'Thou shalt not bear false witness'" (*Human Cloning and Embryonic Stem Cell Research,* 2006). For Doerflinger, the scientific fraud produced by Hwang Woo-Suk in South Korea is the logical consequence of utility-based ethics that ignores the embryo's personhood. While this argument makes reference to embryology, it differs from Doerflinger's arguments in congressional hearings prior to Bush's speech. It treats the scientific observation as secondary to the moral considerations at work in his testimony. The problem with utilitarian ethics for Doerflinger is that it violates moral claims that define embryos as human life deserving respect and protection.

President Bush also eschews a scientistic idiom for an argument grounded in morality when he announces his veto of the 2006 Stem Cell Research Enhancement Act. He shares the stage with a number of children, who were originally adopted when they were embryos. While he speaks, these children embody the moral claim he makes for opposing expanded ES cell research:

> Yet we must also remember that embryonic stem cells come from human embryos that are destroyed for their cells. Each of these human embryos is a unique human life with inherent dignity and matchless value. We see that value in the children who are with us today. Each of these children began his or her life as a frozen embryo that was created for in vitro fertilization, but remained unused after the fertility treatments were complete. Each of these children was adopted while still an embryo, and has been blessed with the chance to grow up in a loving family.
>
> These boys and girls are not spare parts. *(Applause.)* They remind us of that [*sic*] is lost when embryos are destroyed in the name of research. They remind us that we all begin our lives as a small collection of cells. And they remind us that in our zeal for new treatments and cures, America must never abandon our fundamental morals. (Bush, 2006)

Bush's statement reiterates the claim about embryo adoption first presented by opponents in mid-2001: Embryos frozen after IVF can be adopted by infertile couples, thus meaning that no embryo is "spare" or "left over." This claim is ultimately grounded in the series logic extending personhood to all embryos, but while Bush briefly references the scientistic idiom with his recognition that all people start "as a small collection of cells," the claim is grounded in America's "fundamental morals" that require recognition of the embryo's "inherent dignity and matchless value."

In addition to presenting their claims in a moralistic language rather than a scientistic idiom, opponents of ES cell research frame the overall argument as one of science and religion opposed to each other. This frame is presented during the 2004 election by First Lady Laura Bush. During an interview, she cautions, "We have to be really careful between what we want to do for science and what we should do ethically. And stem-cell issue [*sic*] is certainly one of those issues that we need to treat very carefully" ("Laura Bush Advises," 2004). Richard Doerflinger provides a similar contrast when he depicts a "new" utilitarian ethic of science—which he claims is a cover for allowing science to run amok—

versus the "old ethic" that respects human life and accords it inherent value (*Human Cloning and Embryonic Stem Cell Research,* 2006). This strategy can also be seen in the opening of Bush's announcement of the veto of the Stem Cell Research Enhancement Act, when he claims, "In this new era, our challenge is to harness the power of science to ease human suffering without sanctioning the practices that violate the dignity of human life" (Bush, 2006). Whether they present the issue as a challenge that requires caution or the result of scientific arrogance and immorality, opponents frame the debate as one of science versus morality.

The presentation of ES cell research as a struggle between science and religiously based moral sentiment is amplified in the media. In many articles, journalists portray a struggle between science and religion by placing antithetical statements side by side. This is especially common in stories during the 2004 and 2006 elections ("Coming This Week," 2006; "Stem Cell Debate," 2004; "Stem Cell Research Hot Campaign Topic," 2004; Stolberg, 2006a; "Where the Presidential Candidates," 2004). In addition to the placement of opposing sources and their remarks, many news reports make this contrast explicit. A 2005 story on a bill to expand ES cell research began, "A new CBS poll found that 58 percent of those surveyed approve using embryonic stem cells in medical research. That's up from 50 percent just last summer, but opponents, including the president, see this as akin to abortion" ("House Republicans Join Democrats," 2005). A *New York Times* article describing the creation of induced pluripotent cells observes, "Embryonic stem cells are attractive to scientists because they have the potential to grow into any cell or tissue in the body and could, theoretically, be used to treat many ailments. Opponents, including Christian conservatives, say it is immoral to destroy embryos to obtain cells" (Stolberg, 2007). Some journalists report the division between opponents and proponents, while others amplify the situation with language depicting strife. In the conclusion to his report on stem cell research and cloning, Wyatt Andrews observes, "What's coming in Congress is a major battle between morality and science, the scientific belief these microscopic embryos are the fountain of youth against the belief that embryos should not be biofactories" ("Recent Advances in Human Cloning," 2004). A 2006 article describes the Senate's passage of the Stem Cell Research Enhancement Act as a "showdown" with President Bush, which represents the most recent chapter in a debate that "has yielded a complex collision of politics, religion and science since 1998" (Stolberg, 2006b). Another article from that year describes the situation as a "showdown" and warns, "Expect to witness a debate about science and morality" (Skiba, 2006). The organization of news stories builds on viewpoints that describe science and religion at odds over ES cell research: Science becomes increasingly presented as facts without values, while religion becomes values without facts. Such perceptions are amplified by the language connoting strife.

This oppositional framing makes sense for journalists, who turn to conflict to generate interest in a story. Besides journalists, opponents of ES cell research are most likely to turn to this way of framing the issue. It creates the perception that the only values-driven position in the debate is the oppositional view grounded in concerns about abortion and the potential life of the embryo. It attempts to take advantage of proponents' continued use of a scientistic idiom in which the ideological and value-based commitments are implicit assumptions rather than explicit statements. Such perceptions also dovetail with commonplace depictions of scientists as amoral Dr. Frankensteins who fail to recognize the dangers in violating a moral order that inheres in nature (Mulkay, 1996).

Returning to a Scientistic Idiom

Manichean idioms of the ES cell debate present science as opposed to ethics and thus empty of normative values. The claims about an amoral science are encouraged by explicit statements by scientists differentiating science from religion. Additionally, the values driving proponents' arguments—and most scientistic arguments—operate implicitly since the goal of the scientistic idiom they use is to transform their ideological and value commitments into the taken-for-granted assumptions of a debate. While an explicit frame of science versus religion could harm causes that use a scientistic idiom, that antagonistic frame does not harm proponents in the ES cell debate for two reasons. First, proponents continue to reiterate appeals to application, as noted earlier, and for the most part succeed in defining stem cells as the best means to medical applications: Their appeal, which embodies a commitment to helping the sick, becomes *the* primary definition of ES cells. Second, proponents begin to describe the arguments by opponents as explicitly ideological, as part of a partisan political agenda. Most attempts at redefining opposition to ES cell research were abbreviated and first appeared during the 2004 election. In an NBC news segment "In His Own Words," Dr. Irving Weissman claimed, "We are stuck with an ideological ban of this kind of research" ("Dr. Irving Weissman," 2004). Another news report noted that John Kerry "accuses the President of putting ideology before science" ("Stem Cell Research Hot Campaign Topic," 2004). In both cases, the word "ideology" is used instead of "morality." The commonplace understanding of the term connotes self-interested political deception, but the term equally implies that the attitudes defined as "ideological" run counter to the general concern for all people implied by "ethics" or "morality" *and* that it runs counter to the ideal of scientific "objectivity." Both readings are possible, and the selection of one over the other will reflect the attitudes of individual readers and viewers—whether they feel that the moral stance of ES cell opponents masks some underlying ethical hypocrisy or whether they feel that the concerns of opponents run counter to objective standards for truth and knowledge.

Except for brief remarks like these, this argument by (re)definition remains undeveloped until March 2009, when President Barack Obama unveiled an executive order expanding stem cell research and a memorandum calling for the protection of scientific inquiry. As part of that announcement, Obama dismisses the claims of opponents as both a minority point of view out of step with the opinion of the majority and a point of view propped up by lies about ES cell research justified by "ideological" motives. Obama's speech treats these ideological motivations not as denials of scientific objectivity but as arguments running counter to the "natural" order of American ideological commitments. His argument moves through three steps.

First, Obama reiterates the real definition of ES cells as the best means toward achieving medical applications. He says, "At this moment, the full promise of stem cell research remains unknown, and it should not be overstated. But scientists believe these tiny cells may have the potential to help us understand, and possibly cure, some of our most devastating diseases and conditions" (Obama, 2009, para. 2).[5] Even as he warns against overstating the potential of the research and reiterates that much "remains unknown," Obama indicates that ES cells promise to help us understand or cure a variety of diseases. Yet, achieving those ends requires hard work and government support: "But that potential will not reveal itself on its own. Medical miracles do not happen simply by accident. They result from painstaking and costly research—from years of lonely trial and error, much of which never bears fruit—and from a government willing to support that work" (para. 3). The potential of ES cells will only be realized by the lonely labor of scientists supported by the government. The failure to provide that support means that, according to Obama, "promising avenues go unexplored" (para. 3). Obama reiterates these points later in his remarks: "Ultimately, I cannot guarantee that we will find the treatments and cures we seek. No President can promise that. But I can promise that we will seek them—actively, responsibly, and with the urgency required to make up for lost ground" (para. 8). Obama blends the promise of scientific research with a presidential promise of action. While the promise—the *kairos* of medical and scientific possibilities opened up by ES cell research—is controlled by technological and scientific advances beyond our control, Obama associates that promise with the commitment to seek potential medical applications through federal support for ES cell research.

Second, Obama attacks views of science and morality as antagonistic, and he blames that viewpoint for the lack of progress in ES cell research: "But in recent years, when it comes to stem cell research, rather than furthering discovery, our government has forced what I believe is a false choice between sound science and moral values. In this case, I believe the two are not inconsistent. . . . I believe we have been given the capacity and will to pursue this research—and the humanity and conscience to do so responsibly" (para. 4). For Obama, presenting ES cell research as a battleground between science and morality is a forced and false choice. While Obama understands the concerns opponents have about ES cell research (para. 5), he argues, "The proper course has become clear. The majority of Americans—from across the political spectrum, and of all backgrounds and beliefs—have come to a consensus that we should support this research" (para. 6).

While concerns about ES cell research are understandable, the false choice of science or religion is not. Obama associates this false choice about ES cell research with the broader issue of protecting scientific inquiry: "This Order is an important step in advancing the cause of science in America. But let's be clear: Promoting science isn't just about providing resources—it is also about protecting free and open inquiry. . . . It is about ensuring that scientific data is never distorted or concealed to serve a political agenda—*and that we make scientific decisions based on facts, not ideology*" (para. 10; emphasis mine). In order to make sure scientific decisions are based on facts, Obama instructs the White House Office of Science and Technology Policy to develop ways to promote scientific integrity in policy decisions. He does this to ensure that "we base our public policies on the soundest science; that we appoint scientific advisors based on their credentials and their experience, not their politics or ideology" (para. 12).

Obama exposes the false dichotomy of science versus religion and calls for additional funding for this research "to make up for lost ground." Yet, he says, the failure of the previous administration to fund ES cell research properly is only one way in which the government harmed scientific progress. Ideology, Obama implies, had trumped facts, and political coercion had impeded scientific inquiry and progress.[6] In addition to expanding funding for ES cell research, Obama professes to return facts to their proper place in creating government policy. On one level, Obama replicates the impossible self-image of science as utterly disinterested inquiry. As countless scholars have shown time and again, science has always been *interested* inquiry, influenced by ideological and political issues. Yet, to judge Obama as being duped by science's idealized image overlooks how "ideology" is used in Obama's speech. Over the course of the speech, "ideology" becomes associated with the partisan concerns of different political groups. Such partisan concerns fail to discern how the process of limiting the influence of political parties and political appointees serves a broader agenda, which Obama highlights in the final component of his argument.

Third, Obama articulates a vision of America and its values that becomes the ultimate term for adjudicating between different scientific and political proposals: "America"—with all the typical political connotations of patriotism and superiority in technological, but also moral, matters—becomes the ultimate term that adjudicates between the partisan dialectical terms "faith" and "science."[7] Science becomes valuable because of its contribution to the common good and its contribution to America's dominant position in world affairs. Opposition to science becomes "ideological" insofar as it impedes the realization of this vision.

This vision of America's technological and scientific dominance appears at the beginning of Obama's remarks. He notes that his administration will lift the ban on ES cell research, and then says, "And we will aim for America to lead the world in the discoveries it one day may yield" (para. 1). The role of government in helping scientists realize medical miracles offers an inspiring image: "From life-saving vaccines, to pioneering cancer treatments, to the sequencing of the human genome—that is the story of scientific progress in America" (para. 3). This capsule history highlights the successes of government-supported science in the United States, and this string of successes implies that government support for ES cell research will lead to similarly groundbreaking discoveries and inventions.

While scientific advances can be a source of patriotic pride and technological dominance, they also support the common good—understood here as health and absence of disease—for all people. This is apparent in two of the successes of government-supported research, vaccines and cancer treatments, but it also appears in the principle driving studies of ES cells. Obama states, "As a person of faith, I believe we are called to care for each other and work to ease human suffering" (para. 4). This statement does two things. First, it inoculates Obama's viewpoint from claims trying to reiterate a science-versus-religion frame: His faith "calls" him to care for those who are sick and to seek cures for their ailments. Second, while he prefaces this as a religious remark, the belief in easing suffering is universal, embodied in the support communities will provide to those who experience a tragedy, as well as implied in the Constitution's call to "promote the general welfare." In other words, Obama's ostensibly religious sentiment has non-religious and American connotations.

Obama's call to protect scientific inquiry also supports America's technological preeminence: "By doing this, we will ensure America's continued global leadership in scientific discoveries and technological breakthroughs. That is essential not only for our economic prosperity, but for the progress of all humanity" (para. 11). It also protects the well-being of the American people. According to Obama, "[Protecting scientific inquiry] is how we will harness the power of science to achieve our goals—to preserve our environment and protect our national security; to create the jobs of the future, and live longer, healthier lives" (para. 12). Protecting scientific inquiry from interference by political appointees and operatives looking to benefit their party or patrons becomes the key to fulfilling American desires for national security, jobs, health, and the environment.

Obama's speech refutes the framing of the ES cell debate as one of science combating religion and returns to the scientistic idiom. He uses real definitions of ES cells focused on medical applications and ties that research to broader American desires for preeminence in all fields, including science and technology, for healthier lives, and for a way to ease the suffering of the sickest among us. He casts the science-versus-religion frame as a false dichotomy, and while he never explicitly identifies it as ideological, the structure and tone of his remarks associate that false dichotomy with the ideological manipulation of science. Here, "ideology" becomes the cynical manipulation of science and fact *not* because it disturbs the purity of a disinterested or objective science. Manipulation of science becomes ideological because it puts the interests of a political party over American interests. ES cell research and science generally are valuable because they comport with American values, interests, and desires, and in this case, those desires and interests are portrayed as the very best components of the American self-image: a view of America as a leader in all fields whose works ultimately benefit all American citizens and all the world's peoples.

Conclusion

On August 9, 2001, President Bush inserted himself into the debate on ES cell research. His speech offered a qualified "yes" to questions about whether ES cell research should go forward and announced a policy that allowed researchers to use federal money to support that research. Yet, in weighing the relative merits of supporting and opposing ES cell research, Bush portrays ES cells as *both* a way to save a life and a way of taking away an unborn life, rendering any decision incoherent. This combination occurred in part because Bush's presentation of the two sides placed them in a state of near-equilibrium and also because this Manichean idiom, unlike a scientistic idiom, presented the opposing sides as irredeemably tied to science or to morality and religion. The use of a science-versus-religion frame made identifying grounds for a coherent policy impossible, and a balanced presentation did not allow Bush or his listeners to identify a clear winning side whose advice should be followed.

Following President Bush's speech, discourse about ES cells reiterated the definitions used by Bush and those who preceded him. Science tried to realize the promise of stem cells and find research pathways that avoided raising opponents' abortion-based objections. Public discourse reiterated the promise of medical applications and concerns about the embryo, and it often presented the debate as one of science versus morality. While it was sometimes portrayed as scientists versus Catholics and abortion foes, or Democrat versus pro-life Republican, some political discourse presented the conflict as essential to the very nature of science and morality: Scientists would overreach unless moral people united and prevented immoral research.

There were a few attempts to undo this frame, primarily during the 2004 election, but these reached their apotheosis with President Obama's remarks on ES cell research and scientific inquiry. Science versus morality presents a false dichotomy and is associated with manipulations of scientific inquiry and scientific findings. Obama describes this as ideological, and while that terminology comports with idealized views of science, that ideological leaning is a result of some advocates failing to comport their rhetoric with American values. Obama praises science, calls for its protection, and promises to use the best science in crafting policy because doing so comports with American ideological commitments. Science provides medical miracles and other technological innovations that can be used to improve American lives and also secure the nation's preeminence in a given arena, thus playing to patriotic sentiments while also allowing American scientists and corporations to make a profit. While the future of political discourse is hard to predict, Obama has managed to reinforce definitions of ES cells by their potential applications and weld that definition to a vision of American ideals that includes American preeminence in technology and the improved health and welfare of American citizens.

Scientistic and Manichean Idioms of Public Argument

Rhetorical scholars have identified a variety of idioms, modes, styles, and fashions in public argument. This multiplicity finds its genesis in the variety of issues publics must address and in the interactions of the individuals, social movements, and political concerns that constitute those publics. From 1998 through 2001, anti-abortion foes, patient advocates, scientists, feminists, environmentalists, celebrities, and the usual swarm of politicians, pundits, and lobbyists engaged in a vigorous debate about ES cell research, and that debate would flare up after 2001 with the announcement of additional scientific breakthroughs and during the 2004, 2006, and 2008 elections. The breadth and extent of this debate highlight the increased role scientific issues play in the public sphere. As a result, idioms of public argument—unique configurations of substantive and stylistic devices—for handling scientific issues have arisen. Two of those modes, the ones that appeared prominently in debates about ES cell research, are the scientistic idiom and the Manichean idiom. This concluding chapter will draw out the implications of these modes of public argument about science, and it will also highlight the lessons to be drawn about the rhetorical practice of definition and the interaction of scientific and public discourse.

Scientistic Idioms

Public argument co-opts a wide variety of scientific and quasi-scientific language as it grapples with issues raised by scientific research and development. I describe this co-optation or borrowing of scientific language as a *scientistic* idiom in order to recognize its linkage to the rhetoric used in science as well as its discrete existence. In borrowing keywords, arguments, and stylistic figures from science, the scientistic idiom performs two basic functions: It creates "real definitions," quasi-stable points from which individuals can launch arguments that aim to shape our view of the world and direct action, and it aligns those real definitions with American ideological commitments, including freedom, support of community, the general welfare, a general pragmatic outlook, and so on. Given the variety of rhetorical forms used to link these "real definitions" and these ideological commitments, it is more accurate to talk about *variations* of the scientistic idiom or *multiple* scientific idioms: Since the language of biomedicine differs from the languages of physics and chemistry, attempts at fashioning a scientistic idiom from the resources of each scientific discipline will involve different rhetorical styles and vocabulary. Scientistic idioms borrow language and concepts from scientific rhetoric, but their language is more than quasi-scientific, which implies bad science regurgitated by an ignorant public and requiring continual revision by a scientific cognoscenti. Rather, while scientistic idioms depend on scientific rhetoric and practice as a source of invention, they operate in the public sphere independently of scientific control. Scientists might intervene in these public debates, with varying degrees of success, but this does not prevent nonscientific publics from using these idioms, even if scientists attempt to discredit the language and arguments being used.

The scientistic idiom addressing ES cell research developed around three central definitional issues. First, individuals within the debate defined ES cell research by its potential ends, the applications that would be discovered through the means of this research. These definitions took hypothetical conjectures about the ends of research and transformed them into levers for producing social action, thus moving the rock of policy using the fulcrum of American desires: the desire to ease the suffering caused by illness, the desire for scientific progress in certain areas, and a desire for the technological and economic superiority that scientific progress brings. ES cell research was defined as the most advantageous and timeliest means to achieve a better understanding of embryonic development, to develop new ways to test pharmaceuticals, and to produce cures and treatments for diseases for which no treatment currently exists. Second, individuals defined ES cells by their point of origin—spare embryos—and turned to scientific language about "species" and references to the human DNA shared by embryos and born persons to fortify objections to ES cell research. Many, but not all, opponents of this research defined ES cells as an embryo or the murder of an unborn child. Journalists portrayed the debate as an extension of the broader abortion debate, even as a number of prominent pro-life politicians publicly supported the research. Proponents redefined the category "embryo" either to carve out an exception in the form of "spare embryos" that would never result in children or to create two new categories—"pre-embryos" and "embryos"—where the former category consisted of objects scientists could use legitimately to derive ES cells. Finally, individuals in the debate organized the various types of stem cells into a hierarchy by linking them to specific levels of "potency," specific capacities to differentiate and become multiple types of cells. This hierarchy and its ambiguities were loosely tethered to scientific uses of those terms. Scientists and nonscientists would try to modify the perceived "distance" between scientific arguments about hierarchy and public arguments about hierarchy: Scientists tried to minimize the perceived distance in order to constrain the scientific idiom, while nonscientists usually increased perceptions of difference in order to liberate the scientistic idiom and the capacity to use the rhetoric of science independently of scientific control. At stake was the ability to argue in political and journalistic arenas for one of three conclusions: Adult stem cells represented a viable approach to medical applications; ES cells alone were capable of the full range of medical applications; or the science was uncertain, and research in both areas must go forward.

Definition in Science-Focused Debates

The ES cell debate and the three definitional issues central to it highlight the rhetorical nature of definition. When people try to persuade others, definition plays a central role: To the degree that a definition predominates in a debate, then the position predicated on that definition will be predominant to the same degree. Yet these definitions are not clearly stated like a major premise of an Aristotelian syllogism; they rarely appear prominently, as Weaver's claims about argument *from* definition imply (Weaver, 1952). In fact, explicit dependence on a definition or definitions almost always will lead to argument *about* definition and a potentially fruitless wrangle over which definition is most fitting for the situation (Schiappa, 1993). Individuals tend to engage in argument *by* definition when "the key definitional move is simply stipulated, as if it were a natural step along the way of justifying some other claim" (Zarefsky, 1998, p. 5). Acts of definition do not present themselves as definition. Rather, the conceptual point, which becomes the fulcrum of an argument with which a rhetor would shift an entire debate, appears as a relatively innocuous statement. Definitions of ES cells as pluripotent in the scientific literature appear as part of a description of human development, and rhetors do not place particular emphasis on this one point above the others surrounding it. Much of the oppositional discourse extending personhood to the embryo uses phrases like "live embryos" and "unborn children" as a natural and unremarkable part of the discourse. Highlighting definitions is synthetic, the act of critics trying to identify the key assumptions and concepts shaping a debate yet not entirely apparent in the flow of the textual moment. Because definition so often occurs as a matter-of-fact process, it does not take a set form. Various formal rhetorical strategies might be employed in defining a concept. In the ES cell debate, *kairos,* the creation of a series or *incrementum,* hierarchy–based arguments, and references to scene (that is, the abortion debate as ground or scene for ES cell debates) all play a role in defining what ES cells and ES cell research are.

This also reinforces the fact that rhetorical definition is almost always an act of *partial* definition. Each of the three types of strategies used in defining ES cells focuses on one component of what ES cells are—a means to an end, the derivative of a blastocyst, and one type of cell among a variety of cells with similar capacities. While many rhetorical acts incorporate all three types of definition, it is not necessary for any rhetorical act to do so. The articles that first announced the derivation of human ES cells did not address origin and the moral concerns about the embryo or place these cells in a hierarchical relationship with other cell types. Some opposition rhetoric focused almost entirely on the origin of ES cells—how their derivation was the murder of an unborn child—without addressing application or their relation to other cells. Various combinations of these three types of definition are possible, and within each strategy, a whole host of specific definitional tactics exist that might be used separate from the others. When proponents attack claims that ES cells are the murder of developing life, there are multiple avenues of response, but with the exception of Arthur Caplan's testimony in 1998, almost none of the attempts at redefining the issue incorporate all the avenues of response. When individual rhetors highlight the possible applications that ES cell research will produce, only scientists consistently address all three applications, and only a handful of scientists and non-scientists turn to metaphor. Multiple modes of definition exist. That multiplicity results in choice, and out of that choice comes the partiality of any definition.

The partiality of definition also highlights the fact that all acts of definition, all rhetorical discourse, are fragmentary. As Michael McGee (1999) argues, "The apparently finished discourse is in fact a dense reconstruction of all the bits of other discourses from which it is made. It is fashioned from what we can call 'fragments'" (p. 70). Definitions are components—fragments—folded into a larger discourse. These definitional fragments can be collected together by the critic into a "complete" definition, but this whole is not predetermined or intrinsically necessary. The three types of definitions discussed in this book offer a "complete" definition insofar as they are the most prevalent strategies in this stage of the debate, and a "complete" definition, as I use the term here, does not necessarily represent an exhaustive catalog or description of every possible or actual rhetorical strategy. Rather, it is a selection of discursive fragments, but that selection is reflective of the issues and pragmatic concerns driving the debate at a given point in time. Change the debate and the pragmatic concerns from medical applications to issues surrounding biotechnology and intellectual property, and "stem cells" will be defined in relation to patents, licensing arrangements, and material transfer agreements.[1] If you consider the debate about "stem cells" that occurred prior to the isolation of ES cells, "stem cells" would have been defined in relation to "germ plasm" or the regenerative capacities of animals like the hydra (Cooper, 2003; Ramalho-Santos & Willenbring, 2007). Calling a definition "complete" is a function of the debate within which that definition is articulated.

The issue of completeness also highlights the issues of realism: To what extent do words reflect reality, and to what extent do they play a more constitutive role? Many scholars have argued against naïve realism and views of language as primarily a representation of reality that animated earlier discussions of definition, like those found in Richard Weaver's writing (1952). Arguments that ES cells are "really" the best path toward a cure for diabetes or that ES cells are "really" more potent than adult stem cells are not exemplars of naïve realism. Scholars of rhetoric should understand these "real" definitions as a psychosocial consensus by a group of language users. What counts as "real" will change with different groups and will change within groups over time. In fact, "reality" is a quasi-stable point, the intersection of our consensus in language use and action, and the point where that consensus encounters both the recalcitrance and enabling capacities of material objects.

Ideology, Values, and Translation

The "reality" established by definition presents itself as facts. Yet as Ulrich Beck has argued, facts could be different insofar as they are answers to questions that could have been asked differently. These definitions move through various arenas of discourse and action. In that movement, there is a process of translation: As nonscientists take up scientific concepts and products, the forms in which these ideas are communicated change to emphasize the value for a broader society. Previous accounts of translation were limited, and the biggest limitation has been the failure to address the role of persuasion in contrast to structural or economic factors. Specifically, previous accounts do not address how the public comes to accept certain facts over others when each side of a scientific debate has equivalent access to the media, financial resources, social capital, and such. The acceptance of one version of the "facts" presented by a group rather than the perspective and "facts" of another group occurs because scientistic idioms make definitions comport with public ideological commitments. A definition comports with those commitments when it presents a reality—a set of "facts"—wherein the interests of a given public can be furthered. The sheer amount of scientific work published, along with its complexity and its sometimes contradictory findings, produces a range of options for individual partisans and groups who then select facts that support their point of view. These partisan uses of science could undermine science's standing and its ability to produce facts: Science could appear to be a mere tool of biased parties. Yet two things mitigate this possibility. First, scientists are not passive: They try to maintain control over their discursive resources and insulate themselves from some public uses of their work. Second, scientistic idioms move beyond partisan, dialectical appeals and present definitions so they comport with the ultimate, or overarching, ideological values of a community or collective.

This drive to align the definitions produced in science and the already existing commitments of a public means there is less divergence in values than has been implied by some studies of science-public interaction. This examination of the ES cell debate has highlighted the similarity in values motivating scientists and nonscientists. Ultimately, both groups value ES cell research for pragmatic reasons, and a main motivator for both groups is the possibility of medical applications. This highlights the desire to improve human life, as well as "baser" motives such as fame for finding or supporting the research that led to a new medical application and the financial benefits to groups that make such a discovery. Even the differences in motivation—the fact that scientists additionally desire research and pharmaceutical applications from ES cell research—highlight the pragmatic orientation of both groups. Scientists pursue ES cell research because of the ends that it can help them achieve, not for a chaste, value-neutral, epistemic goal of accruing knowledge for the sake of knowledge.

In this case, the values shaping the desired end goals are embodied in definition. Because definitions help establish our "reality" as part of making a consensus on action and language use possible, they always embody value judgments. At the most basic level, definition indicates that a given issue or object deserves attention: It should be selected and made a figure against the backdrop of other objects, issues, and actions. This pragmatic orientation encompasses scientific and nonscientific definition, meaning we should continue questioning claims that science is value neutral. While rhetoricians of science have made this point repeatedly, it deserves repetition here because of how supporters of science and ES cell research have responded to Manichean framings of science.

Manichean Idioms

The Manichean idiom frames issues as a struggle between science and some opponent, usually religion or morality, and it involves attempts at diminishing the credibility of one's opponents. It has been well researched in relation to attempts by scientists to enlarge their share of social resources and epistemic authority at the expense of other intellectual traditions, like religion and the humanities (Ceccarelli, 2001; Lessl, 1996, 2007). In those cases, scientists claim religion has hampered human development and happiness or that the humanities and social sciences try to plumb the depths of human nature with crude tools in contrast to physical science's elegant and expensive equipment. Yet, a parallel Manichean idiom appears in concerns that scientists are creating Frankenstein's monster or leading us to a brave new world (Mulkay, 1996; The President's Council on Bioethics, 2002, chapter 6; 2004, pp. 93–94).

It is this latter version of the idiom—religion defending the ramparts of culture against the invasion of amoral science—that circulates most frequently in the ES cell debate. The dichotomy of science and religion at the heart of this idiom works to forestall scientific progress. The idiom eliminates anything but an antagonistic relationship between the two: While some people using a Manichean idiom will try to balance the desire for the fruits of science with caution, they still portray nonscientists as a group that must approach science cautiously and continually fear that using science will lead to the unraveling of their most closely held values (for a further example of this rhetoric, see The President's Council on Bioethics, 2002). The benefits of science may be acknowledged, but science itself will be at best grudgingly accepted. In many situations in which the Manichean idiom has appeared, even grudging acceptance is not possible. This is best illustrated by the debates about teaching evolution in public schools. Here, supporters of intelligent design and creationism aim to prevent further elaboration of science and evolution in classrooms and hope to establish educational policies that lead to their theory (intelligent design or creationism) being taught.[2]

In addition to stymieing scientific endeavors and education, a Manichean idiom could also make it easier to misuse and abuse science: If science cannot be trusted to provide "appropriate" tools and facts, it might become more acceptable to manipulate science and produce one's own facts, as the Bush administration did with its censoring of scientific reports and selective use of research for its own ends. Subsequent to the abuse of science by the Bush administration, many people have reiterated calls for a "value-neutral" science, one free from partisan influence or somehow independent from politics (see, for example, "Dr. Irving Weissman," 2004; Mooney, 2006).[3] Such visions also turn to a Manichean idiom, although one presenting science as the force for good. Generally, hype and conflict, like that surrounding the ES cell debate, can make greater amounts of information available and lead to increased public engagement with issues (Nisbet & Huge, 2006; Olien, Donohue, & Tichenor, 1995; Wilcox, 2003), but such conflict—if it is to produce effective public engagement—must allow for the perception or creation of alternatives and compromises that can be circulated in interpersonal, journalistic, and public contexts. With a Manichean idiom, conflict has been rendered so extreme that compromise is no longer possible. A Manichean idiom will still animate groups, but it leads to acrimony and divisiveness, resulting in a stalemate between religion, science, and politics. That stalemate became embodied in President Bush's stem cell policy.

Moving Forward in Science-Policy Debates

From 1998 to 2001, the United States experienced a vigorous debate about research on embryonic stem cells. The debate became heated as it moved across scientific, political, and journalistic arenas, but it was often conducted in a scientistic idiom that required shaping the appeals made and definitions offered so they comported with American ideological commitments, ranging from freedom and opportunity to the pragmatic and the desire to support others in need (whether those in "need" were defined as patients or as embryos). In 2001, George W. Bush inserted himself into the debate and transformed it by speaking in a Manichean idiom that depicted scientific privateering that threatened to undermine the (religious) values and ideals of society. While such a worldview had been used in journalistic coverage of the opposition prior to August 2001 and might have been used by opponents of ES cell research in some cases, the majority of the political discourse used a scientistic idiom. After Bush's speech, more political and policy discourse turned to a Manichean idiom. President Obama undercut the Manichean idiom and claimed it offered a false dichotomy to Americans, but it is still not clear whether the scientistic idiom will return to the fore of public argument about stem cells.

By now, it is evident that I prefer the scientistic idiom to the Manichean idiom. The scientistic idiom provides a way to incorporate the findings of science into public argument, as well as providing a rhetorical mechanism for establishing the "facts" or "reality" of a situation. It is preferable to a Manichean idiom for at least two reasons. First, the scientistic idiom is available to any public speaker, regardless of his or her affiliation with science. As can be seen from the ES cell debate, scientists, ethicists, politicians, and people from different religious backgrounds have employed it. While the opponents of ES cell research "lost" both when President Bush authorized limited ES cell research and when President Obama expanded that research, it was because their primary objection to ES cell research—that it destroys human embryos—requires people to believe embryos are fully equivalent to an actual born person. The attitudes people have toward embryonic life are complex, and depend in part on an emotional identification with fetuses that is attenuated in the ES cell debate. That attenuation occurs because the embryos from which the cells are derived are not visibly human. In addition to this limitation, advocates of ES cell research were effective in defining ES cells as a cure for common afflictions. Given that opponents also understood stem cells generally as a means to produce medical applications, one should not be surprised that advocates of ES cell research carried the day.

Second, the Manichean idiom grinds down the complexities of an issue so that it fits simple us-versus-them categories. While less extreme conflicts can lead to greater information and public engagement, the conflict of a Manichean idiom ultimately harms the quality of information and engagement. Moving toward a more nuanced understanding of what values science embodies and supports has the potential to move public argument past the impasse and division that result from a Manichean idiom. Scientific activity will never replace ethics and religion, but by understanding the ethical and moral component of scientific practices, we can better integrate the two. Many concerns about scientific practice are driven by the perception that science has no respect for communal values or restraint: The image of out-of-control and amoral science becomes a less powerful anti-scientific line of argument when the values motivating scientists become apparent. A scientistic idiom does not necessarily lead to a better understanding of scientific research, but it can make the values driving that research intelligible insofar as they exist in the translation of scientific rhetoric and practice into a scientistic idiom.

In the case of ES cell research, an understanding of the moral underpinnings of pro–ES cell positions could help move the debate forward and provide lay publics the means to grapple with developments in science. The goal of medical applications embodies a moral precept of medical science—providing help to the ill. Care for others is the basis for much of our moral code, and pretending that the ES cell research issue is one of amoral science versus moral and religious objections obfuscates the complex ethical issues in the debate. Recognizing this moral value embedded in the research would help people fruitfully engage in public deliberation on this issue. One can imagine a situation in which discussion of medical applications of new research is not met with claims that the science is being "oversold" for the nefarious purposes of researchers but rather the discussion moves to the relative costs and benefits of seeking cures via this research avenue. Furthermore, while the full technical complexity of ES cell derivation, maintenance, and differentiation will elude many people, this does not mean that lay people do not, or will not, understand the basics of ES cell research. Research has shown that lay people understand the basics of mutation and the issues surrounding genetic technology and that their judgments about these areas differ from those of scientists because of the value judgments they have made (Bates, Lynch, Bevan, & Condit, 2005; Condit, Dubriwny, Lynch, & Parrott, 2004). Defining the policy options for ES cell research in terms of the values represented by opponents *and* proponents would allow for greater and more fruitful public deliberation on this issue. Ideally, such a move could shape many public debates about biotechnology.

Notes

Chapter 1

1. By *naïve* realism, I mean a commonsense view that the ultimate or essential constituents of the world can be explicated and that language provides direct access to that reality. For rhetorical examinations of *philosophical realism,* see Schiappa (1993, pp. 409–412) and Gross (1990, pp. 193–207).

2. Beck's book *Risk Society: Towards a New Modernity* describes the shift over the last 50 years from a modern society concerned with the production and distribution of wealth to a risk society with a reflexive and systematic concern for managing the risks produced by modern life. Beck argues that modern, industrial society undergoes a "reflexive modernization" that results in the disruption of the logic of wealth distribution because it is forced to compete with the logic of risk distribution. For him, science plays two roles in the risk society: First, science is the simultaneous cause and solution of various risks (e.g., nuclear accidents like Chernobyl result from deploying knowledge of physics, while those same studies contribute to attempts at controlling and remediating the results of those accidents), and second, the authority of science becomes diffused throughout society, becoming available to a greater number of people and interest groups. It is the qualities of contemporary science described by Beck, especially the latter quality, that I draw upon in characterizing debates about stem cell research and the scientistic idiom.

3. By emphasizing that the "primary" framing is religion versus science, I foreground the public attitudes represented in surveys like those from 2007 and 2009 showing that one-third of Americans believe that human beings have not evolved and a majority believe that a divine power was involved in humanity's creation (Keeter, Smith, & Masci, 2007; Pew Research Center, 2009). I am not making claims here about the conceptual underpinnings of intelligent design (ID), which has tried to shape religious beliefs about creationism into a scientific theory. The rhetorical contours of ID have been studied elsewhere (Campbell & Meyer, 2003).

4. While many discussions of science's ideologies use the term "scientism," Weaver's discussion of scientific ideologies uses the term "scientistic" (Weaver, 1970).

5. All scientific discourse analyzed within this book was identified using a snowball method. I began with scientific review articles on stem cell research. Articles mentioned in the first layer—in more than one scientific review article—became part of the

"second layer," and articles mentioned in two or more of the research articles became the "third layer" of the sample. This method found a core of 50 review and research articles that scientists cited presenting work at the nexus of the debate about embryonic and adult stem cells.

Congressional testimony was accessed using LEXIS-NEXIS Congressional, using an advanced search of all hearings with the term "stem cell" appearing anywhere in the hearing. When PDF documents of hearings are available, page numbers for pertinent quotations are provided.

Journalistic discourse came from two sources. First, the Vanderbilt Television News Archive was used to identify 103 television news stories that addressed stem cell research. The sample from 1998 to 2002 included material from ABC, CBS, CNN, and NBC, while the sample from 2004 onward also included FOX News. Second, the newspaper articles examined came from a two-tiered sample. A two-tiered sample was used in order to gather discourse from the most prominent newspaper sources in America as well as to gather a breadth of the discourse used across the United States. The first tier consists of high-impact papers, specifically *The New York Times* and *USA Today.* They represent the most prominent U.S. newspaper and the most popular U.S. newspaper. The second tier consists of low-impact papers, consisting of newspapers from various cities throughout the United States. Both samples were collected through LEXIS-NEXIS news search, and each tier consists of 100 news articles in order to maintain a manageable amount of discourse to be studied.

Key terms were identified by using a basic text search, and a term was identified as key to the definition of stem cell if it appeared in four or more sources in a given body of discourse (i.e., if a term was found four times in scientific discourse, it was identified as part of the scientific definition; if a term was found four times in Congressional discourse, it was identified as part of the political definition, etc.). Descriptive statistics were developed for each body of discourse, and rhetorical methods of analysis were used to identify the definitional patterns into which the terms were organized.

Chapter 2

1. While using a concept over 2,000 years old to explain current technological and scientific developments appears questionable on its face, Miller (1994) argues that this application is necessary and valuable. The development of a technology, like the move of stem cell research from the laboratory bench to the hospital bedside, involves the same need for reasoned action in the face of uncertainty that characterizes the issues of war, taxes, etc., that were the bailiwick of classical rhetoric.

2. For more on the sampling methods used, see chapter 1, note 5.

3. This does not mean that capitalist motives are absent from the discourse, just that they are not prominent. When journalist accounts deal with business, they focus on the value of stem cell research for the biotech industry (Allison, 2001; Brister, 2001; Epstein, 2000; Krantz, 2001; Pollack, 2001a, 2001b), while the political discussion of business-related issues typically focuses on patents (*Stem Cell Research,* 1999; *Stem Cells 2001,* 2001).

4. In addition to Varmus's broad claim of stem cell application, Dr. Thomas Okarma of Geron Corporation made similar claims about the potential of embryonic stem cells to "usher in a new era of therapeutic opportunities" (*Stem Cell Research*, 1999, p. 59).

Chapter 3

1. This is not a statement about the state of biological science, but rather an issue of perception. Some scientists argue that evolutionary theory is necessary to understand any contemporary advance in biology (see, e.g., Miller, 2008; Zimmer, 2001). That said, the practice of creating new medical cures and technologies is not obviously linked to evolution in public discourse.

2. A similar move is made in the journalistic observation that abortion opponents view ES cell research as the same as murder (Connolly, Gillis, & Weiss, 2001; Mishra, 2001b, 2001c).

3. The circulation of newspaper stories describing the various religious and ethical stands on ES cell research would also provide audiences a way to conceive of the research as being "pro-life" (Ackerman, 2001; "Dealing with Hard Ethical Questions," 2000; "Embryo Research Debated," 1998; Friend, 2001b; Olson, 2000a; Zitner, 1999).

4. See the prepared testimonies of Andrew Kimbrell from the International Center for Technology Assessment, an environmental advocacy group, and Judy Norsigian of the Boston Women's Health Book Collective (*Dangers of Cloning*, 2002).

5. Laury Oaks (2000) reaches a similar conclusion: "Representations of fetuses as persons and patients are unlikely to fade given legal attempts to recognize fetal rights, the development of medical treatments for fetuses, and the fact that many women experience and think of their babies-to-be as specific individuals" (p. 67).

6. While not focusing on the effects of fetal surgery, many feminist scholars have addressed the discursive creation of mother-fetus antagonism. A sample of these works includes: Duden, 1993; Morgan, 1996; Morgan & Michaels, 1999; Rothman, 1989; Spallone, 1989; Stabile, 1994.

7. "Respect" is used here in an uncritical fashion that does not consider ways in which technological intervention could be "respectful" while still resulting in the risk of destruction. François Baylis (2001) argues that this uncritical use also appears in key documents about the ethics of ES cell research.

8. The same situation holds in Great Britain where death certificates are not produced for miscarriages before 20 weeks of gestation (Williams et al., 2001).

9. Embryoid bodies are collections of ES or EG cells that have been left to transform into a variety of specialized cell types. While these bodies have shown some organization of tissue-like muscle, skin, and nerve cells, no researcher has ever reported that these groups of cells simultaneously produced all the cell types in an embryo or recapitulated the development of an embryo.

10. Similar phrasing appears in Dooley, 2001; Hall, 2001; Hesman, 2001b; Vergano, 2001b; and Wade, 2001a.

11. Similar remarks can be found in "Controversy Surrounding," 2001.

Chapter 4

1. For more on "fragments" and "fragmentation" as a theory of discourse and rhetoric, see M. C. McGee, 1999.

2. The "enthymeme" is an argument in which the audience participates by providing the premises left unstated by the rhetor (see Johnstone, 2001).

3. Reeve's question was incorporated into an NBC news report ("Christopher Reeve Asks," 2000).

4. Hatch's comment is also aired as part of CNN's coverage of the stem cell debate ("Stem Cell Research," 2001).

Chapter 5

1. Fahnestock argues that the visual element of repetition exists also in the use of graphic elements in scientific argument, as well as in the use of words.

2. Two sources do explicitly define the term "multipotency" as the ability to produce all the cells of a specific tissue type, such as the epithelium or the cells of the blood (Slack, 2000; van der Kooy & Weiss, 2000).

3. A recent glossary on the terminology of stem cell research offers the term "oligopotent" to describe lesser degrees of multipotency. "Multipotency" refers to cells that "can form multiple lineages that constitute an entire tissue," while "oligopotency" refers to the ability to form two cell types (Smith, 2006, p. 1060).

4. Some individuals also identify ES cells as "totipotent" (Clarke et al., 2000; Weissman, 2000a, 2000b), but the association of totipotency with embryonic stem cells is not widespread and has been criticized as confusing embryonic stem cells with more primitive (and powerful) cells like the fertilized egg (Smith, 2001).

5. This placement also reaffirms the argument that ES cells are not embryos, discussed in chapter 3.

6. The one exception to this trend appears in a December 18, 2001, *New York Times* story providing a retrospective on stem cell research in 2001. This story presents the hierarchy of cell types but uses the metaphor of chess pieces to describe them: ES cells are the queen who "can perform all the permissible moves," while adult stem cells are bishops, knights, and rooks who can perform a limited set of moves, and fully mature cells are pawns with only one role (Wade, 2001b).

7. The study is by Petersen and colleagues (see Petersen et al., 1999). For similar arguments by this journalist, see Srikameswaran, 1999b, 2000.

Chapter 6

1. All subsequent citations in the text will be to paragraphs of President Bush's August 9, 2001, speech.

2. This remark comes from Senator Specter's prepared testimony. It was in a set of HTML full-text documents containing testimony from the hearing, which was available

from 2002 to 2005, but it was not included in the final version of the hearing transcript currently available in the LEXIS-NEXIS Congressional database.

3. See note 2 regarding source information for Senator Specter's testimony.

4. Johnson makes a similar remark in a 2006 newspaper article on congressional attempts to expand ES cell research (Skiba, 2006).

5. All subsequent citations in the text will be to paragraphs of President Obama's March 2009 speech.

6. Numerous definitions of ideology exist, but almost all would agree that modern science is implicated in the extant ideologies shaping the contemporary world and, for some, that science has its own unique ideology. For more on ideology and its various definitions, see Eagleton, 1991, especially chapter 1; Williams, 1983, pp. 153–157.

7. Burke describes three terms for order: positive, dialectical, and ultimate. Positive terms refer to objects. Dialectical terms deal with motives and ideals, and each of these motives exists in tension with each other, unless they are adjudicated by ultimate terms that provide the basis for evaluating different motives and placing them within a hierarchy. Ultimate terms help organize the motives driving people and help individuals adjudicate between various motives. (Burke, 1969a, pp. 183–189)

Chapter 7

1. Issues of patents are discussed during the period under examination; they were the focus of a meeting of the Senate Appropriations subcommittee on Labor, Health and Human Services and Education in January 1999 (*Stem Cell Research,* 1999). Yet, patents do not come to the forefront of the public debate, which focused more on the relative morality of helping future patients through ES cell research versus harming potential lives by deriving ES cells.

2. While the Supreme Court has ruled that creation science represents an undue imposition of religion by the state, groups like Answers in Genesis, which built and runs the Creation Museum in Petersburg, Kentucky, still advocate for creationism.

3. The Bush administration engaged in a number of actions to shape science for its political and ideological ends. Political appointees at the FDA overruled recommendations of staff scientists and advisory panels that Plan B emergency contraception be approved for over-the-counter use. The Bush administration and its appointees also rewrote scientific reports and public documents and censored what scientists could say: For example, a National Cancer Institute fact sheet was altered in 2003 to claim there was a link between abortion and breast cancer, which does not exist, and White House staff would edit the work of climate scientists to downplay the risk of global warming. See Dean, 2007; Marquis, 2003; Mooney, 2006, 2007; Shulman 2006.

Works Cited

Abate, T. (2000, April 24). Hearings on stem cell research just the start of long debate. *The San Francisco Chronicle,* p. B1.

Ackerman, T. (2001, July 8). Hopes high for stem-cell solution. *The Houston Chronicle,* p. A2.

Ackerman, T., & Roth, B. (2001, August 11). In stem cell debate, what comes next? Some scientists dubious of Bush-approved plan. *The Houston Chronicle,* p. A1.

Actor and research advocate Christopher Reeve dies at age of 52. (2004). New York: CBS News.

Allison, W. (2001, July 30). Mixing business with science. *St. Petersburg Times,* p. 1A.

Amit, M., Carpenter, M. K., Inokuma, M. S., Chiu, C.-P., Harris, C. P., Waknitz, M. A., et al. (2000). Clonally derived human embryonic stem cell lines maintain pluripotency and proliferative potential for prolonged periods of culture. *Developmental Biology, 227*(2), 271–278.

Asen, R. (2009). Ideology, materiality and counterpublicity: William E. Simon and the rise of the conservative counterintelligentsia. *Quarterly Journal of Speech, 95,* 263–288.

Associated Press. (1998, December 3). Experts say ban on embryo study slows research. *St. Louis Post-Dispatch,* p. A12.

Associated Press. (1999, January 22). Experiment suggests way to grow new organs; patient's own cells would be used to make tissues. *St. Louis Post-Dispatch,* p. A8.

Bates, B. R., Lynch, J. A., Bevan, J. L., & Condit, C. M. (2005). Warranted concerns, warranted outlooks: A focus group study of public opinion about genetics research. *Social Science and Medicine, 60,* 331–344.

Baylis, F. (2001). Human embryonic stem cell research: Comments on the NBAC report. In S. Holland, K. Labacqz, & L. Zoloth (Eds.), *The human embryonic stem cell debate: Science, ethics, and public policy* (pp. 51–60). Cambridge, MA: MIT Press.

Beck, U. (1992). *Risk society: Towards a new modernity.* London: Sage Publications.

Bjornson, C. R., Rietze, R. L., Reynolds, B. A., Magli, M. C., & Vescovi, A. L. (1999). Turning brain into blood: A hematopoietic fate adopted by adult neural stem cells in vivo. *Science, 283*(5401), 534–538.

Bloomberg News. (2009, August 19). Study using embryonic stem cells is delayed. *The New York Times,* p. B8.

Bookman, J. (2001, July 8). Divided over stem cells; the escalating debate over the poten-

tial of using human embryos in treating a variety of diseases pits medical researchers against right-to-life groups. *The Atlanta Journal-Constitution*, p. 1D.

Boyd, J. (2002). Public and technical interdependence: Regulatory controversy, out-law
discourse, and the messy case of Olestra. *Argumentation and Advocacy 39*, 91–109.

Brave new world cloning humans. (2004). New York: ABC News.

Brister, K. (2001, October 24). Stem cell lab wrestles with questions; OK for federal
funding no guarantee of success for Athens-based BresaGen. *The Atlanta Journal-
Constitution*, p. 5E.

Brown, D. (2001, August 12). Stem cell decision examined; scientists are wondering
about its impact on their work. *The Washington Post*, p. A8.

Bucchi, M. (1998). *Science and the media: Alternative routes in scientific communication*. London: Routledge.

Burke, K. (1966). *Language as symbolic action: Essays on life, literature, and method*. Berkeley:
University of California Press.

Burke, K. (1969a). *A grammar of motives*. Berkeley, CA: University of California Press.

Burke, K. (1969b). *A rhetoric of motives*. Berkeley: University of California Press.

Bush defends decision. (2001). Atlanta: CNN News.

Bush talks about stem cell research and Middle East while on vacation. (2001). New
York: NBC News.

Bush, G. W. (2001). Remarks by the president on stem cell research. Retrieved April 6,
2004, from http://www.whitehouse.gov/news/releases/2001/08/20010809-2.html.

Bush, G. W. (2006). President discusses stem cell research policy. Retrieved March 15,
2007, from http://www.whitehouse.gov/news/releases/2006/07/20060719-3.html.

Bush's stem cell decision proves divisive. (2001). Atlanta: CNN News.

Cadavers are latest source of versatile stem cells. (2000, November 6). *The Washington
Post*, p. A19.

Campbell, J. A., & Meyer, S. C. (Eds.). (2003). *Darwinism, design, and public education*. East
Lansing: Michigan State University Press.

Campbell, J. E. (2004). The 2000 presidential election of George W. Bush: The difficult
birth of a presidency. In J. Kraus, K. J. McMahon, & D. M. Rankin (Eds.), *Transformed by crisis: The presidency of George W. Bush and American politics* (pp. 9–28). New
York: Palgrave MacMillan.

Casper, M. (1998). *The making of the unborn patient: A social anatomy of fetal surgery*. [Elec-
tronic Version]. New Brunswick, NJ: Rutgers University Press.

Ceccarelli, L. (2001). *Shaping science with rhetoric*. Chicago: Chicago University Press.

Centers for Disease Control. (2004). Fetal death, *NCHS data definitions*.

Christopher Reeve asks Congress to allow federal funds for stem cell research. (2000).
New York: NBC News.

Christopher Reeve remembered for his role as research advocate. (2004). New York:
CBS News.

Chung, Y., Klimanskaya, I., Becker, S., Marh, J., Lu, S.-J., Johnson, J., et al. (2006). Embryonic and extraembryonic stem cell lines derived from single mouse blastomeres.
Nature, 439(7073), 216–219.

Clarke, D. L., Johansson, O. B., Wilbertz, J., Veress, B., Nilsson, E., Karlstrom, H., et al. (2000). Generalized potential of adult neural stem cells. *Science, 288*(5471), 1660–1663.

Cloning, 2001, special hearing: Hearings before the Subcommittee on Labor, Health and Human Services, and Education, of the Senate Appropriations Committee, 107th Cong., 1 (2001).

Cloning, 2002, special hearings: Hearings before the Subcommittee on Labor, Health and Human Services, and Education, of the Senate Appropriations Committee, 107th Cong., 2 (2002).

Cohen, C. (2007). *Renewing the stuff of life: Stem cells, ethics, and public policy.* Oxford: Oxford University Press.

Collins, H. M. (1992). *Changing order: Replication and induction in scientific practice.* Chicago: University of Chicago Press.

Coming this week . . . a stem-cell showdown. (2006, July 16). *The Atlanta Journal-Constitution,* p. 1C.

Complication in President Bush's policy regarding the federal funding of stem cell research. (2001). New York: CBS News.

Condit, C. M. (1990). *Decoding abortion rhetoric: Communicating social change.* Chicago: University of Illinois Press.

Condit, C. M., Dubriwny, T. N., Lynch, J. A., & Parrott, R. L. (2004). Lay people's understandings of and preference against the term "mutation." *American Journal of Medical Genetics, 130A,* 245–250.

Congress debates embryonic stem cell research. (2001). New York: CBS News.

Connolly, C., Gillis, J., & Weiss, R. (2001, August 20). Viability of stem cell plan doubted; Bush policy could limit research, scientists say. *The Washington Post,* p. A1.

Controversy brewing over embryonic stem cell research. (2001). New York: CBS News.

Controversy over stem cell research. (2000). New York: ABC News.

Controversy surrounding stem cell research (2001). New York: NBC News.

Cook, G. (2006, August 24). Stem-cell method preserves embryo. *The Boston Globe,* p. A1.

Cooper, M. (2003). Rediscovering the immortal *hydra:* Stem cells and the question of epigenesis. *Configurations, 11,* 1–26.

Cowan, C. A., Klimanskaya, I., McMahon, J., Atienza, J., Witmyer, J., Zucker, J. P., et al. (2004). Derivation of embryonic stem-cell lines from human blastocysts. *New England Journal of Medicine, 350,* 1353–1356.

Curtis, R. (1994). Narrative form and normative force: Baconian story-telling in popular science. *Social Studies of Science, 24,* 419–461.

Daley, G. Q. (2004). Missed opportunities for embryonic stem-cell research. *New England Journal of Medicine, 351,* 627–628.

D'Amour, K. A., Bang, A. G., Eliazer, S., Kelly, O. G., Agulnick, A. D., Smart, N. G., et al. (2006). Production of pancreatic hormone-expressing endocrine cells from human embryonic stem cells. *Nature Biotechnology, 24*(11), 1392–1401.

Dangers of cloning and the promise of regenerative medicine: Hearings before the Senate Committee on Health, Education, Labor and Pensions, 107th Cong., 2 (2002).

Daniels, J. T., Dart, J. K., Tuft, S. J., & Khaw, P. T. (2001). Corneal stem cells in review. *Wound repair and regeneration: Official publication of the wound healing society [and] the European tissue repair society, 9*(6), 483–494.

D.C. police search Gary Condit's home, looking for clues to the whereabouts of Chandra Levy. (2001). On *Wolf Blitzer Reports*. Atlanta: CNN.

Dealing with hard ethical questions as stem cell research accelerates. (2000, August 28). *Tampa Tribune,* p. 8.

Dean, C. (2007, January 31). Scientists criticize White House stance on climate change findings. *The New York Times,* p. A17.

Debate in White House over controversial stem cell research. (2001). New York: ABC News.

Debate over embryonic stem cell research (2001). New York: CBS News.

Debate over President Bush's stem cell research funding decision. (2001). New York: CBS News.

Debate over stem cell research (2001). New York: NBC News.

Dooley, T. (2001, August 4). There's no consensus on stem-cell research. *The Houston Chronicle,* p. 1.

Doyle, R. (1997). *On beyond living: Rhetorical transformations of the life sciences.* Stanford, CA: Stanford University Press.

Dr. Irving Weissman on stem cell research. (2004). New York: NBC News.

Dr. Tim Johnson explains what exactly stem cells do and what the research would be used for. (2001). New York: ABC News.

Drazen, J. (2004). Embryonic stem-cell research—the case for federal funding. *New England Journal of Medicine, 351,* 1789–1790.

Duden, B. (1993). *Disembodying women: Perspectives on pregnancy and the unborn.* Cambridge, MA: Harvard University Press.

Eagleton, T. (1991). *Ideology: An introduction.* London: Verso.

Embryo research debated; battle rages as cells grow in lab. (1998, November 15). *Chicago Sun-Times,* p. 43.

Embryonic stem cell research. (2001). New York: CBS News.

Embryos created for stem cell research only. (2001). New York: ABC News.

Enormous scientific breakthrough. (1998). New York: ABC News.

Epstein, B. (2000, August 23). Banking on stem cells. *St. Petersburg Times,* p. 4D.

Evans, M. J., & Kaufman, M. H. (1981). Establishment in culture of pluripotential cells from mouse embryos. *Nature, 292*(5819), 154–156.

Exploring the promise of embryonic stem cell research: Hearing before the Special Committee on Aging, United States Senate, 109th Cong., 1 (2005).

Fabj, V., & Sobnosky, M. J. (1995). AIDS activism and the rejuvenation of the public sphere. *Argumentation and Advocacy, 31,* 163–185.

Fahnestock, J. (1993). Accommodating science: The rhetorical life of scientific facts. In M. W. McRae (Ed.), *The literature of science: Perspectives on popular scientific writing* (pp. 17–36). Athens: University of Georgia Press.

Fahnestock, J. (1999). *Rhetorical figures in science.* Oxford: Oxford University Press.

Farrell, T. B., & Goodnight, G. T. (1981). Accidental rhetoric: The root metaphors of Three Mile Island. *Communication Monographs, 48,* 271–300.

Federal guidelines for stem cell research revive debate on whether or not possible medical advances outweigh any ethical concerns. (2000). New York: CBS News.

Ferrari, G., Cusella-DeAngelis, G., Coletta, M., Paolucci, E., Stornaiuolo, A., Cossu, G., et al. (1998). Muscle regeneration by bone marrow–derived myogenic progenitors. *Science, 279*(5356), 1528–1530.

Fletcher, J. C. (2001). The stem cell debate in historical context. In S. Holland, K. Labacqz, & L. Zoloth (Eds.), *The human embryonic stem cell debate: Science, ethics, and public policy* (pp. 27–34). Cambridge, MA: MIT Press.

Fox, C. (2007). *Cell of cells: The global race to capture and control the stem cell.* New York: W. W. Norton & Co.

Franklin, S. (1999). "Orphaned" embryos. In J. Edwards, S. Franklin, E. Hirsch, F. Price & M. Strathern (Eds.), *Technologies of procreation: Kinship in the age of assisted conception* (2nd ed.). New York: Routledge.

Friend, T. (1999, May 24). OK to fetal tissue research may ignite ethical firestorm. *USA Today,* p. 1A.

Friend, T. (2000, May 7). Stem-cell study regenerates enthusiasm. *USA Today,* p. 9D.

Friend, T. (2001a, July 12). Debate intensifies over stem cell research. *USA Today,* p. 10D.

Friend, T. (2001b, July 19). From tiny cells, large life issues. *USA Today,* p. 8D.

Friend, T. (2001c, August 28). Labs chosen to give USA stem-cell lines. *USA Today,* p. 3A.

Friend, T. (2001d, August 10). Scientists predict huge impact on human life. *USA Today,* p. 5A.

Friend, T. (2001e, August 8). Stem-cell debate mixes science, religion, politics. *USA Today,* p. 7A.

Friend, T. (2001f, July 17). The stem cell hard sell. *USA Today,* p. 6D.

Friend, T. (2001g, August 21). Stem-cell talks aim to iron out ethical, legal issues. *USA Today,* p. 5D.

Friend, T. (2001h, May 7). Stem-cell study regenerates enthusiasm. *USA Today,* p. 9D.

Frum, D. (2003). *The right man: The surprise presidency of George W. Bush.* New York: Random House.

Gage, F. H. (2000). Mammalian neural stem cells. *Science, 287*(5457), 1433–1438.

Gardner, R. L., & Beddington, R. S. P. (1988). Multi-lineage "stem" cells in the mammalian embryo. *Journal of Cell Science Supplement, 10,* 11–27.

Gearhart, J., Pashos, E. E., & Prasad, M. K. (2007). Pluripotency redux—advances in stem-cell research. *New England Journal of Medicine, 357*(15), 1469–1472.

George Bush visits Pope John Paul II and discusses embryonic stem cell research (2001). New York: NBC News.

Gieryn, T. (1983). Boundary-work and the demarcation of science from non-science: Strains and interests in professional ideologies of scientists. *American Sociological Review, 48,* 781–795.

Gilbert, C., & Skiba, K. M. (2001, June 17). Thompson in the thick of things on stem cell research funding debate. *Milwaukee Journal Sentinel,* p. 9A.

Gillis, J., & Connolly, C. (2001, August 24). Stem cell research faces FDA hurdle. *The Washington Post*, p. A1.

Goldstein, A., & Allen, M. (2001, August 10). Bush backs partial stem cell funding. *The Washington Post*, p. A01.

Goodell, M. A., Brose, K., Paradis, G., Conner, A. S., & Mulligan, R. C. (1996). Isolation and functional properties of murine hematopoietic stem cells that are replicating in vivo. *Journal of Experimental Medicine, 183*(4), 1797–1806.

Goodnight, G. T. (1982). The personal, technical, and public spheres of argument: A speculative inquiry into the art of public deliberation. *Journal of the American Forensic Association, 18,* 214–227.

Goodwin, D. (1991). Distinction, argumentation, and the rhetorical construction of the real. *Argumentation and Advocacy, 27,* 141–158.

Gross, A. G. (1990). *The rhetoric of science.* Cambridge, MA: Harvard University Press.

Guthrie, P. (2001, August 10). The process may open door to medical miracles; but reliance on embryos controversial. *The Atlanta Journal-Constitution*, p. 10A.

Hall, C. T. (2000, November 6). Promising way to repair brain. *The San Francisco Chronicle*, p. A1.

Hall, C. T. (2001, July 23). Seeds of possibility; the debate over using stem cells harvested from embryos has been complicated by the discovery that adult stem cells are found throughout the human body. *The San Francisco Chronicle*, p. A4.

Hartouni, V. (1997). *Cultural conceptions: On reproductive technologies and the remaking of life.* Minneapolis: University of Minnesota Press.

Hawhee, D. (2004). *Bodily arts: Rhetoric and athletics in ancient Greece.* Austin: University of Texas Press.

Haybron, R. (1999, May 2). Stem cell research may someday stem suffering. *Plain Dealer*, p. 9K.

Health officials pinpoint stem cell lines that researchers can use and have federal tax dollars pay for it. (2001). New York: CBS News.

Here's what debate on stem cells is all about. (2001, August 10). *The Seattle Times*, p. A2.

Herold, E. (2006). *Stem cell wars: Inside stories from the frontlines.* New York: Palgrave Macmillan.

Hesman, T. (2000, August 24). New policy eases research on embryo cells. *St. Louis Post-Dispatch*, p. A1.

Hesman, T. (2001a, April 22). Promise of stem cell research collides with ethics, politics. *St. Louis Post-Dispatch*, p. A1.

Hesman, T. (2001b, July 15). Scientists worry about power vacuum. *St. Louis Post-Dispatch*, p. B1.

Highly controversial new advances in human cloning science. (2004). New York: NBC News.

Hilliard, B., Lansford, T., & Watson, R. P. (Eds.). (2004). *George W. Bush: Evaluating the president at midterm.* Albany: State University of New York Press.

Holland, S., Lebacqz, K., & Zoloth, L. (Eds.). (2001). *The human embryonic stem cell debate: Science, ethics, and public policy.* Cambridge, MA: MIT Press.

House Republicans join Democrats to pass legislation clearing the way for stem-cell research. (2005). New York: CBS News.

Hult, K. M., & Walcott, C. E. (2007). Early evaluations of the Bush presidency. *Rhetoric and Public Affairs, 10,* 361–370.

Human Cloning: Hearing before the Subcommittee on Science, Technology and Space of the Committee on Commerce, Science and Transportation, United States Senate, 107th Cong., 1 (2001).

Human cloning and embryonic stem cell research after Seoul: Examination, exploitation, fraud and ethical problems in the research: Hearing before the Subcommittee on Criminal Justice, Drug Policy and Human Resources of the Committee on Government Reform, House of Representatives, 109th Cong., 2 (2006).

Hwang, W. S., Ryu, Y. J., Park, J. H., Park, E. S., Lee, E. G., Koo, J. M., et al. (2004). Evidence of a pluripotent human embryonic stem cell line derived from a cloned blastocyst. *Science, 303,* 1669–1674.

Influential Senator Bill Frist gives a boost to supporters of embryonic stem cell research (2001). New York: CBS News.

Inside story: Hollywood and stem cell research. (2004). New York: CBS News.

Institute of Medicine. (2002). *Stem cells and the future of regenerative medicine.* Washington DC: National Academies Press.

The International Stem Cell Initiative. (2007). Characterization of human embryonic stem cell lines by the International Stem Cell initiative. *Nature Biotechnology, 25,* 803–816.

Irwin, A. (2001). Constructing the scientific citizen: Science and democracy in the biosciences. *Public Understanding of Science, 10*(1), 1–18.

Jackson, K. A., Majka, S. M., Wang, H., Pocius, J., Hartley, C. J., Majesky, M. W., et al. (2001). Regeneration of ischemic cardiac muscle and vascular endothelium by adult stem cells. *Journal of Clinical Investigation, 107*(11), 1395–1402.

Jackson, K. A., Mi, T., & Goodell, M. A. (1999). Hematopoietic potential of stem cells isolated from murine skeletal muscle. *Proceedings of the National Academy of Sciences of the United States of America, 96*(25), 14482–14486.

Johnson, D. (2006). Dawkins' myth: The religious dimensions of evolutionary discourse. *Journal of Communication and Religion, 29,* 285–314.

Johnson, D. (2008). Psychiatric power: The post-museum as a site of rhetorical alignment. *Communication and Critical/Cultural Studies, 5,* 344–362.

Johnstone, C. L. (2001). Enthymeme. In *Encyclopedia of Rhetoric.* New York: Oxford University Press.

Jones Institute recruits volunteers to donate eggs and sperm for controversial stem cell research (2001). New York: NBC News.

Jordan, C. T., Guzman, M. L., & Noble, M. (2006). Cancer stem cells. *New England Journal of Medicine, 355,* 1253–1261.

Joss, S., & Durant, J. (Eds.). (1995). *Public participation in science: The role of consensus conferences in Europe.* London: Science Museum.

Keen, J., & Welch, W. M. (2001, July 18). Bush faces agonizing choice; stem-cell debate mixes ethics, emotions, politics and progress. *USA Today,* p. 8A.

Keeter, S., Smith, G., & Masci, D. (2007). *Religious belief and public attitudes about science in the U.S.* Washington, DC: Pew Research Center.

Keller, E. F. (2002). *Making sense of life: Explaining biological development with models, metaphors, and machines.* London: Harvard University Press.

Keränen, L. (2005). Mapping misconduct: Demarcating legitimate science from "fraud" in the B-06 lumpectomy controversy. *Argumentation and Advocacy, 42,* 94–113.

Kiely, K. (2001a, September 11). Broader stem-cell research sought. *USA Today,* p. 1A.

Kiely, K. (2001b, August 10). Bush's decision moves the debate to Congress. *USA Today,* p. 6A.

Kiely, K., & Hall, M. (2001, August 8). Stem-cell debate hits home for lawmakers. *USA Today,* p. 1A.

King, W. (1999, January 21). Seattle scientist's stem-cell research shows promise for humans. *The Seattle Times,* p. B3.

King, W. (2001, August 20). High on the future: Already saving lives, stem-cell research may soon be in full swing. *The Seattle Times,* p. A1.

Kirtley, B. (2004). The arbiter of fate: The presidential character of George W. Bush. In B. Hilliard, T. Lansford, & R. P. Watson (Eds.), *George W. Bush: Evaluating the president at midterm* (pp. 19–28). Albany: State University of New York Press.

Kolata, G. (2001, December 18). The stem cell debate: A thick line between theory and therapy, as shown with mice. *The New York Times,* p. F3.

Krantz, M. (2001, September 6). Stem cells not drawing cash. *USA Today,* p. 3B.

Kraus, J., McMahon, K. J., & Rankin, D. M. (Eds.). (2004). *Transformed by crisis: The presidency of George W. Bush and American politics.* New York: Palgrave MacMillan.

Lagasse, E., Connors, H., Al-Dhalimy, M., Reitsma, M., Dohse, M., Osborne, L., et al. (2000). Purified hematopoietic stem cells can differentiate into hepatocytes *in vivo. Nature Medicine, 6*(11), 1229–1235.

Landmark in embryo research complicates stem cell debate. (2001). Atlanta: CNN News.

Latour, B. (1987). *Science in action: How to follow scientists and engineers through society.* Cambridge, MA: Harvard University Press.

Latour, B., & Woolgar, S. (1986). *Laboratory life: The construction of scientific facts* (2nd ed.). Princeton, NJ: Princeton University Press.

Laura Bush advises caution regarding stem cell research (2004). New York: CBS News.

Leach, M., & Scoones, I. (2005). Science and citizenship in a global context. In M. Leach, I. Scoones, & B. Wynne (Eds.), *Science and citizens: Globalization and the challenge of engagement* (pp. 15–38). London: Zed Books.

Lengner, C. J., Camargo, F. D., Hochedlinger, K., Welstead, G. G., Zaidi, S., Gokhale, S., et al. (2007). *Oct4* expression is not required for mouse somatic stem cell self-renewal. *Cell Stem Cell, 1,* 403–415.

Leonard, M. (2000, August 24). Abortion foes see politics in stem-cell study policy. *The Boston Globe,* p. A1.

Less stem research available than many first assumed. (2001). New York: NBC News.

Lessl, T. M. (1988). Heresy, orthodoxy and the politics of science. *Quarterly Journal of Speech, 74,* 18–34.

Lessl, T. M. (1996). Naturalizing science: Two episodes in the evolution of a rhetoric of scientism. *Western Journal of Communication, 60,* 379–396.

Lessl, T. M. (1999). The Galileo legend as scientific folklore. *Quarterly Journal of Speech, 85,* 146–168.

Lessl, T. M. (2002). Gnostic scientism and the prohibition of questions. *Rhetoric and Public Affairs, 2,* 133–157.

Lessl, T. M. (2007). The culture of science and the rhetoric of scientism: From Francis Bacon to the Darwin Fish. *Quarterly Journal of Speech, 93,* 123–149.

Limited stem cell research funding sends America's scientists overseas (2001). New York: ABC News.

Lore, D. (2001, September 6). 24 stem-cell lines available for U.S.-funded study. *Columbus Dispatch.*

Lynch, J. A. (2006). Making room for stem cells: Dissociation and establishing new research objects. *Argumentation and Advocacy, 42,* 143–156.

Lynch, J. A. (2009). Articulating scientific practice: Understanding the "gay gene" study as overlapping material, social and rhetorical registers. *Quarterly Journal of Speech, 95,* 435–456.

Lyne, J. (1990). Bio-rhetorics: Moralizing the life sciences. In H. W. Simons (Ed.), *The rhetorical turn: Invention and persuasion in the conduct of inquiry* (pp. 35–57). Chicago: University of Chicago Press.

Lyne, J. (1996). Quantum mechanics, consistency, and the art of rhetoric: Response to Krips. *Cultural Studies, 10,* 115–132.

Manning, A. (2001, August 14). Stem-cell limits questioned. *USA Today,* p. 8D.

Marchione, M. (1998, November 19). Stem cell finding reopens debate on embryo research. *Milwaukee Journal Sentinel,* p. 17.

Marchione, M. (1999, January 20). Stem cell research cleared to get federal funding. *Milwaukee Journal Sentinel,* p. 1.

Marchione, M. (2000, February 25). Journal explores future of stem cell research. *Milwaukee Journal Sentinel,* p. 14A.

Marcotty, J., & Lerner, M. (2002, January 25). Stem cell feat refuels debate. *Star Tribune,* p. 1A.

Marquis, C. (2003, August 8). Bush misuses science data, report says. *The New York Times,* p. A14.

Martin, G. R. (1981). Isolation of a pluripotent cell line from early mouse embryos cultured in medium conditioned by teratocarcinoma stem cells. *Proceedings of the National Academy of Sciences of the United States Of America, 78*(12), 7634–7638.

McCloskey, D. N. (1998). *The rhetoric of economics* (2nd ed.). Madison: University of Wisconsin Press.

McGee, B. R. (1999). The argument from definition revisited: Race and definition in the Progressive Era. *Argumentation and Advocacy, 35,* 141–158.

McGee, M. C. (1999). Text, context, and the fragmentation of contemporary culture. In J. L. Lucaites, C. M. Condit, & S. Caudill (Eds.), *Contemporary rhetorical theory: A reader* (pp. 65–78). New York: Guilford Press.

Meissner, A., & Jaenisch, R. (2006). Generation of nuclear transfer-derived pluripotent ES cells from cloned Cdx2-deficient blastocysts. *Nature, 439*(7073), 212–215.

Meissner, A., Wernig, M., & Jaenisch, R. (2007). Direct reprogramming of genetically unmodified fibroblasts into pluripotent stem cells. *Nature Biotechnology, 25,* 1177–1181.

Mezey, E., Chandross, K. J., Harta, G., Maki, R. A., & McKercher, S. R. (2000). Turning blood into brain: cells bearing neuronal antigens generated in vivo from bone marrow. *Science, 290*(5497), 1779–1782.

Michelle Kiley discusses controversial need for stem cell research to help cure diabetes (2001). New York: ABC News.

Miller, C. R. (1992). *Kairos* in the rhetoric of science. In S. P. Witte, N. Nakadate, & R. D. Cherry (Eds.), *A rhetoric of doing: Essays on written discourse in honor of James L. Kinneavy* (pp. 310–327). Carbondale: Southern Illinois University Press.

Miller, C. R. (1994). Opportunity, opportunism and progress: *Kairos* in the rhetoric of technology. *Argumentation, 8,* 81–96.

Miller, K. R. (2008). *Only a theory: Evolution and the battle for America's soul.* New York: Penguin Books.

Miller, P., & Oleary, T. (1994). The factory as laboratory. *Science in Context, 7*(3), 469–496.

Mishra, R. (2001a, July 3). Fear, politics slow stem-cell work. *The Boston Globe,* p. A1.

Mishra, R. (2001b, August 11). Stem cell grants could begin in January; battles loom on ownership of embryo "lines." *The Boston Globe,* p. A1.

Mishra, R. (2001c, August 21). What can stem cells really do? *The Boston Globe,* p. C1.

Mishra, R. (2002, March 26). Stem cells converted to functioning blood vessels. *The Boston Globe,* p. A5.

Mitaka, T. (2001). Hepatic stem cells: From bone marrow cells to hepatocytes. *Biochemical and Biophysical Research Communications, 281*(1), 1–5.

Mitchell, G. R. (2000). *Strategic deception: Rhetoric, science, and politics in missile defense advocacy.* East Lansing: Michigan State University Press.

Mody, C. C. M. (2005). The sounds of science: Listening to laboratory practice. *Science Technology and Human Values, 30*(2), 175–198.

Mooney, C. (2006). *The Republican war on science.* New York: Basic Books.

Mooney, C. (2007). *Storm world: Hurricanes, politics, and the battle over global warming.* Orlando, FL: Harcourt.

Mooney, C., & Nisbet, M. C. (2005). When coverage of evolution shifts to the political and opinion pages, the scientific context falls away, unravelling Darwin. *Columbia Journalism Review, 44*(3), 31–39.

Moretti, A., Caron, L., Nakano, A., Lam, J. T., Bernshausen, A., Chen, Y., et al. (2006). Multipotent embryonic Is11+ progenitor cells lead to cardiac, smooth muscle, and endothelial cell diversification. *Cell, 127*(6), 1151–1165.

Morgan, L. M. (1996). Fetal relationality in feminist philosophy: An anthropological critique. *Hypatia, 11*(3), 46–70.

Morgan, L. M., & Michaels, M. W. (Eds.). (1999). *Fetal subjects, feminist positions.* Philadelphia: University of Philadelphia Press.

Moscovici, S. (1984). The phenomenon of social representations. In R. Farr & S. Moscovici (Eds.), *Social representations* (pp. 3–69). London: Cambridge University Press.

Most Americans satisfied with president's stem cell decision. (2001). New York: ABC News.

Mulkay, M. (1996). Frankenstein and the debate over embryo research. *Science, Technology and Human Values, 21*(2), 157–176.

Myers, G. (1990). *Writing biology: Texts in the social construction of scientific knowledge.* Madison: University of Wisconsin Press.

Nancy Reagan's battle over stem-cell research. (2004). New York: NBC News.

National Institutes of Health claims there are enough embryonic stem cell lines, others disagree. (2001). New York: ABC News.

National Institutes of Health. (2001). *Stem cells: Scientific progress and future research directions.* Bethesda, MD: National Institutes of Health.

Nelson, B. (2000, June 11). Promising stem-cell work faces fierce opposition. *The Denver Post,* p. A3.

Nelson, J. S., Megill, A., & McCloskey, D. N. (Eds.). (1987). *The rhetoric of the human sciences: Language and argument in scholarship and public affairs.* Madison: University of Wisconsin Press.

New technology to grow new human parts for transplants. (2000). New York: ABC News.

The newshour with Jim Lehrer. (2000, August 24). New York and Washington DC: Public Broadcasting Service.

Nichols, J. (2001). Introducing embryonic stem cells. *Current Biology, 11*(13), R503–R505.

Nichols, J., Zevnik, B., Anastassiadis, K., Niwa, H., Klewe-Nebenius, D., Chambers, I., et al. (1998). Formation of pluripotent stem cells in the mammalian embryo depends on the POU transcription factor Oct4. *Cell, 95,* 379–391.

NIH takes a look at the 60 stem cell lines. (2001). New York: ABC News.

Nisbet, M. C., & Goidel, R. K. (2007). Understanding citizen perceptions of science controversy: Bridging the ethnographic-survey research divide. *Public Understanding of Science, 16,* 421–440.

Nisbet, M. C., & Huge, M. (2006). Attention cycles and frames in the plant biotechnology debate: Managing power and participation through the press/policy connection. *Harvard International Journal of Press/Politics, 11*(2), 3–40.

Oaks, L. (2000). Smoke-filled wombs and fragile fetuses: The social politics of fetal representation. *Signs, 26*(1), 63–108.

Obama, B. (2009). Remarks of President Barack Obama. Retrieved March 9, 2009, from http://www.whitehouse.gov/the_press_office/Remarks-of-the-President-As-Prepared-for-Delivery-Signing-of-Stem-Cell-Executive-Order-and-Scientific-Integrity-Presidential-Memorandum/.

Okita, K., Ichisaka, T., & Yamanaka, S. (2007). Generation of germline-competent induced pluripotent stem cells. *Nature, 448,* 313–317.

Olien, C. N., Donohue, G. A., & Tichenor, P. J. (1995). Conflict, consensus, and public opinion. In T. L. Glasser & C. T. Salmon (Eds.), *Public opinion and the communication of consent* (pp. 301–322). New York: Guilford Press.

Olson, J. (2000a, November 19). Cell research sharply divides Nebraskans. *Omaha World Herald,* p. 1A.

Olson, J. (2000b, August 15). From stem cells to brain cells; discovery doesn't alter NU goal of devising fetal-cell guidelines. *Omaha World Herald,* p. A1.

Olson, J. (2000c, August 24). NU bioethics panel eyes stem-cell research rules. *Omaha World Herald,* p. 8.

Olson, J. (2000d, October 12). NU panel recommends stem-cell guidelines. *Omaha World Herald,* p. 1.

Olson, J. (2000e, September 17). Stem-cell debate picks up. *Omaha World Herald,* p. 1A.

Opportunities and advancements in stem cell research: Hearing before the Subcommittee on Criminal Justice, Drug Policy and Human Resources, of the House Committee on Government Reform, House, 107th Cong., 1 (2001).

Page, S., & Hall, M. (2001, August 10). Compromise may bring flak from both sides. *USA Today,* p. 4A.

Park, I.-H., Arora, N., Huo, H., Maherali, N., Ahfeldt, T., Shimamura, A., et al. (2008). Disease-specific induced pluripotent stem cells. *Cell, 134*(5), 877–886.

Paroske, M. (2009). Deliberating international science policy controversies: Uncertainty and AIDS in South Africa. *Quarterly Journal of Speech, 95,* 148–170.

Partridge, T. (2006). Disciplining the stem cell into myogenesis. *New England Journal of Medicine, 354,* 1844–1845.

Pear, R. (2001, June 27). U.S. study hails stem cells' promise. *The New York Times,* p. A20.

Pearsall, J., & Trumbull, B. E. (2002). *The Oxford English dictionary* (2nd ed., rev. ed.). Oxford: Oxford University Press.

People who are most directly affected by President Bush's decision on funding for stem cell research. (2001). New York: CBS News.

Perelman, C., & Olbrechts-Tyteca, L. (1969). *The new rhetoric.* Notre Dame, IN: University of Notre Dame Press.

Petchesky, R. P. (1990). *Abortion and woman's choice: The state, sexuality, and reproductive freedom.* Boston: Northeastern University Press.

Petersen, B. E., Bowen, W. C., Patrene, K. D., Mars, W. M., Sullivan, A. K., Murase, N., et al. (1999). Bone marrow as a potential source of hepatic oval cells. *Science, 284*(5417), 1168–1170.

Pew Research Center. (2009). *Public praises science; scientists fault public, media.* Washington, DC: Pew Research Center.

Phillips, K. R. (1996). The spaces of public dissension: Reconsidering the public sphere. *Communication Monographs, 63,* 231–248.

Pickering, A. (1984). *Constructing quarks: A sociological history of particle physics.* Edinburgh: Edinburgh University Press.

Pittenger, M. F., Mackay, A. M., Beck, S. C., Jaiswal, R. K., Douglas, R., Mosca, J. D., et al. (1999). Multilineage potential of adult human mesenchymal stem cells. *Science, 284*(5411), 143–147.

Political reaction to President Bush's decision on embryonic stem cell research (2001). New York: NBC News.

Pollack, A. (2000, May 30). Neural cells, grown in labs, raise hopes on brain disease. *The New York Times,* p. F1.

Pollack, A. (2001a, July 28). Another stem cell debate; ethics aside, a good business model remains elusive. *The New York Times,* p. C1.

Pollack, A. (2001b, August 26). The promise in selling stem cells. *The New York Times,* p. C1.

Possibility for private funding when it comes to stem cell research. (2001). New York: ABC News.

President Bush continues vacation; decision on stem cell research awaits his return to the White House tomorrow. (2001). New York: CBS News.

President Bush discusses embryonic stem cell research with Pope John Paul II. (2001). Atlanta: CNN News.

President Bush interviewed about yesterday's stem cell research decision. (2001). New York: ABC News.

President Bush makes decision on federal funding of embryonic stem cell research. (2001). Atlanta: CNN News.

President Bush meets with Pope John Paul II. (2001). New York: ABC News.

President Bush receives lecture from Pope on embryonic stem cell research; rebuke from world leaders about global warming. (2001). New York: CBS News.

President Bush says he will make a decision on federal funding for stem cell research before September. (2001). New York: CBS News.

President Bush supports some federal funding for stem cell research. (2001). New York: CBS News.

President Bush to announce decision on embryonic stem cell research. (2001). New York: NBC News.

President Bush will announce his decision tonight during prime-time TV about federal funding for stem cell research. (2001). New York: ABC News.

President Bush's appeal to Catholic voters. (2001). New York: CBS News.

Presidential ethics panel to explore new genetic technology. (1998). Atlanta: CNN.

The President's Council on Bioethics. (2002). *Human cloning and human dignity: An ethical inquiry.* Washington, DC: Author.

The President's Council on Bioethics. (2004). *Monitoring stem cell research.* Washington, DC: Author.

Ramalho-Santos, M., & Willenbring, H. (2007). On the origin of the term "stem cell." *Cell Stem Cell, 1,* 35–38.

Recent advances in human cloning create major ethical, medical and political concerns. (2004). New York: CBS News.

Research indicates that adult brain stem cells may grow into other tissues, scientists report. (2000, June 2). *St. Louis Post-Dispatch,* p. A9.

Reyes, M., Dudek, A., Jahagirdar, B., Koodie, L., Marker, P. H., & Verfaillie, C. M. (2002). Origin of endothelial progenitors in human postnatal bone marrow. *Journal of Clinical Investigation, 109*(3), 337–346.

Reyes, M., & Verfaillie, C. M. (2001). Characterization of multipotent adult progenitor cells, a subpopulation of mesenchymal stem cells. *Annals of the New York Academy of Sciences, 938,* 231–233.

Rise and fall of South Korea's top scientist. (2005). New York: NBC News.

Rodriguez, P. (2006). Talking brains: A cognitive semantic analysis of an emerging folk neuropsychology. *Public Understanding of Science, 15,* 301–330.

Rothman, B. K. (1989). *Recreating motherhood: Ideology and technology in a patriarchal society.* New York: Viking.

Rushing, J. H., & Frentz, T. (1989). The Frankenstein myth in contemporary cinema. *Critical Studies in Mass Communication, 6,* 61–80.

Saltus, R. (1999, June 8). Hope for repairing brain damage; stem cells in mice are said to migrate to needed areas. *The Boston Globe,* p. A3.

Saltus, R. (2000, July 4). The man who fixes brains. *The Boston Globe,* p. F1.

Schiappa, E. (1985). Dissociation in the arguments of rhetorical theory. *Journal of the American Forensic Association, 22,* 72–82.

Schiappa, E. (1993). Arguing about definitions. *Argumentation, 7,* 403–417.

Schiappa, E. (1996). Towards a pragmatic approach to definition: "Wetlands" and the politics of meaning. In A. Light & E. Katz (Eds.), *Environmental Pragmatism* (pp. 209–230). London: Routledge.

Schiappa, E. (2003). *Defining reality: Definitions and the politics of meaning.* Carbondale: Southern Illinois University Press.

Schmickle, S. (1999a, April 11). Medically tantalizing, ethically wrenching; they might help organs repair themselves or reverse brain damage, but obtaining them from embryos raises the question of whether that constitutes the taking of human life. *Star Tribune,* p. 1A.

Schmickle, S. (1999b, December 17). Stem-cell work named breakthrough of '99: Scientists say the explosion in the understanding of the body's master cells has enormous potential. *Star Tribune,* p. 3A.

Schmickle, S. (2000a, September 14). Politics heats up stem-cell debate. *Star Tribune,* p. 22A.

Schmickle, S. (2000b, November 22). Tapping the master cells. *Star Tribune,* p. 24A.

Schubert, C., & Fauber, J. (2000a, August 24). Rules OK'd for stem cells in U.S.-funded research. *Milwaukee Journal Sentinel,* p. 1A.

Schubert, C., & Fauber, J. (2000b, August 25). Using embryos in study "immoral," Vatican says. *Milwaukee Journal Sentinel,* p. 1B.

Schwartz, R. E., Reyes, M., Koodie, L., Jiang, Y. H., Blackstad, M., Lund, T., et al. (2002). Multipotent adult progenitor cells from bone marrow differentiate into functional hepatocyte-like cells. *Journal of Clinical Investigation, 109*(10), 1291–1302.

Schwartz, R. S. (2006). The politics and promise of stem-cell research. *New England Journal of Medicine, 355,* 1189–1191.

Science/stem cell research. (2000). Atlanta: CNN.

Scientists and anti-abortion activists at odds over the use of stem cell research; President Bush to decide on federal funding soon. (2001). New York: CBS News.

Scott, J. B. (2006). Kairos as indeterminate risk management: The pharmaceutical industry's response to bioterrorism. *Quarterly Journal of Speech, 92,* 115–143.

Seelye, K. Q. (2001, August 10). The President's decision: The overview; Bush gives his backing for limited research on existing stem cells. *The New York Times,* p. A1.

Shamblott, M. J., Axelman, J., Wang, S., Bugg, E. M., Littlefield, J. W., Donovan, P. J., et al. (1998). Derivation of pluripotent stem cells from cultured human primordial germ cells. *Proceedings of the National Academy of Sciences of the United States of America, 95,* 13726–13731.

Shapin, S., & Schaffer, S. (1985). *Leviathan and the air-pump: Hobbes, Boyle, and the experimental life.* Princeton, NJ: Princeton University Press.

Shulman, S. (2006). *Undermining science: Suppression and distortion in the Bush administration.* Berkeley: University of California Press.

Simons, H. W. (Ed.). (1990). *The rhetorical turn: Invention and persuasion in the conduct of inquiry.* Chicago: University of Chicago Press.

Sipiora, P. (2002). Introduction: The ancient concept of *kairos.* In P. Sipiora & J. S. Baumlin (Eds.), *Rhetoric and kairos: Essays in history, theory, and praxis* (pp. 1–22). Albany, NY: State University of New York Press.

Skiba, K. M. (2006, July 16). Showdown set on stem cells: Senate to consider loosening rules. *Milwaukee Journal Sentinel,* p. A1.

Slack, J. M. W. (2000). Stem cells in epithelial tissues. *Science, 287,* 1431–1433.

Smith, A. (2001). Embryo-derived stem cells: Of mice and men. *Annual Review of Cell and Developmental Biology, 17,* 435–462.

Smith, A. (2006). A glossary for stem cell biology. *Nature, 441,* 1060.

Smith, J. E. (2002). Time and qualitative time. In P. Sipiora & J. S. Baumlin (Eds.), *Rhetoric and kairos: Essays in history, theory, and praxis* (pp. 46–57). Albany, NY: State University of New York Press.

Snyder, E. Y., & Loring, J. F. (2006). Beyond fraud—stem-cell research continues. *New England Journal of Medicine, 354,* 321–324.

Solter, D. (2005). Politically correct human embryonic stem cells? *New England Journal of Medicine, 353,* 2321–2323.

Somers, T. (2006, October 20). Novocell says it has manipulated stem cells to fight diabetes. *The San Diego Union-Tribune,* p. C1.

South Korean researchers successfully clone human embryos. (2004). New York: CBS News.

Spallone, P. (1989). *Beyond conception: The new politics of reproduction.* Granby, MA: Bergin & Garvey Publishers.

Spotts, P. N. (2002, February 4). Embryo cloning: Key to stem-cell research? *Christian Science Monitor,* p. 2.

Springer, M. L., Brazelton, T. R., & Blau, H. M. (2001). Not the usual suspects: The unexpected sources of tissue regeneration. *Journal of Clinical Investigation, 107*(11), 1355–1356.

Srikameswaran, A. (1999a, May 14). Bone marrow cells could one day be used to heal damaged livers. *Pittsburgh Post-Gazette,* p. A1.

Srikameswaran, A. (1999b, January 22). Brain cells able to make blood. *Pittsburgh Post-Gazette,* p. A1.

Srikameswaran, A. (2000, September 21). Stem cells can be reprogrammed; they can generate other types of cells. *Pittsburgh Post-Gazette,* p. A5.

Stabile, C. (1994). Shooting the mother: Fetal photograph and the politics of disappearance. In C. Stable (Ed.), *Feminism and the technological fix* (pp. 68–98). Manchester: Manchester University Press.

Stein, R. (2009, January 24). Government approves study using human embryonic stem cells. *The Washington Post,* p. A06.

Stem cell debate: Candidates disagree on issues of research (2004). New York: ABC News.

Stem cell research and patents; funeral for Maureen Reagan. (2001). New York: ABC News.

Stem cell research debate on Capitol Hill (2001). New York: ABC News.

Stem cell research hot campaign topic. (2004). New York: NBC News.

Stem cell research. (2001). *Wolf Blitzer Reports.*. Atlanta: CNN News.

Stem cell research: Hearing before the Committee on Health, Education, Labor and Pensions, 107th Cong., 1 (2001).

Stem cell research, special hearing: Hearings before the Subcommittee on Labor, Health and Human Services, and Education, of the Senate Appropriations Committee, 105th Cong., 2 (1999).

Stem cell research, part 2, special hearing: Hearings before the Subcommittee on Labor, Health and Human Services, and Education, of the Senate Appropriations Committee, 106th Cong., 1 (1999).

Stem cell research, part 3, special hearings: Hearings before the Subcommittee on Labor, Health and Human Services, and Education, of the Senate Appropriations Committee, 106th Cong., 2 (2000).

Stem cells, 2001, special hearing: Hearings before the Senate Committee on Appropriations, Senate, 107th Cong., 1 (2001).

Stolberg, S. G. (2001a, August 17). Patent on human stem cell puts U.S. officials in bind. *The New York Times,* p. A1.

Stolberg, S. G. (2001b, August 10). The president's decision: A question of research; disappointed by limits, scientists doubt estimate of available cell lines. *The New York Times,* p. A17.

Stolberg, S. G. (2001c, January 20). Transition in Washington: Research and morality; stem cell research advocates in limbo. *The New York Times,* p. A17.

Stolberg, S. G. (2006a, April 24). Eyes on November, parties zero in on issues to drive voter turnout. *The New York Times,* p. A1.

Stolberg, S. G. (2006b, July 16). Senate appears poised for a showdown with the president over stem cell research. *The New York Times,* p. A1.

Stolberg, S. G. (2007, November 20). Advance on stem cells equalizes debate. *The New York Times,* p. A23.

Stormer, N. (2000). Prenatal space. *Signs, 26*(1), 109–144.

Supporters of both sides debate over stem cell research. (2001). New York: NBC News.

Tada, M., Takahama, Y., Abe, K., Nakatsuji, N., & Tada, T. (2001). Nuclear reprogramming of somatic cells by in vitro hybridization with ES cells. *Current Biology, 11*(19), 1553–1558.

Takahashi, K., & Yamanaka, S. (2006). Induction of pluripotent stem cells from mouse embryonic and adult fibroblast cultures by defined factors. *Cell, 126*(4), 663–676.

Taylor, C. A. (1996). *Defining science: A rhetoric of demarcation.* Madison: University of Wisconsin Press.

Taylor, C. A., & Condit, C. M. (1988). Objectivity and elites: A creation science trial. *Critical Studies in Mass Communication, 5,* 293–312.

Theise, N. D., Badve, S., Saxena, R., Henegariu, O., Sell, S., Crawford, J. M., et al. (2000). Derivation of hepatocytes from bone marrow cells in mice after radiation-induced myeoablation. *Hepatology, 31*(1), 235–240.

Thomson, J. A., & Odorico, J. S. (2000). Human embryonic stem cell and embryonic germ cell lines. *Trends in Biotechnology, 18*(2), 53–57.

Thomson, J. A., Itskovitz-Eldor, J., Shapiro, S. S., Waknitz, M. A., Swiergiel, J. J., Marshall, V. S., et al. (1998). Embryonic stem cell lines derived from human blastocysts. *Science, 282*(5391), 1145–1147.

Thomson, J. A., Kalishman, J., Golos, T. G., Durning, M., Harris, C. P., Becker, R. A., et al. (1995). Isolation of a primate embryonic stem cell line. *Proceedings of the National Academy of Sciences of the United States of America, 92*(17), 7844–7848.

Titsworth, B. S. (1999). An ideological basis for definition in public argument: A case study of the Individuals with Disabilities in Education Act. *Argumentation and Advocacy, 35,* 171–184.

Tokuzawa, Y., Kaiho, E., Maruyama, M., Takahashi, K., Mitsui, K., Maeda, M., et al. (2003). Fbx15 is a novel target of Oct3/4 but is dispensable for embryonic stem cell self-renewal and mouse development. *Molecular and Cellular Biology, 23*(8), 2699–2708.

Treadway, J. (2002, January 7). Stem cells have varied sources; amid embryo debate, lives saved, prolonged. *Times-Picayune,* p. 1.

US stem cell research steadily losing ground to other nations. (2004). New York: CBS News.

van der Kooy, D., & Weiss, S. (2000). Why stem cells? *Science, 287*(5457), 1439–1441.

Verfaillie, C. M. (2002). Adult stem cells: assessing the case for pluripotency. *Trends in Cell Biology, 12*(11), 502–508.

Vergano, D. (2001a, September 5). Stem cells from Israel are sent to Harvard lab. *USA Today,* p. 2A.

Vergano, D. (2001b, September 6). Thompson: Stem cells not ready. *USA Today,* p. 5A.

Wade, N. (2000a, August 24). New rules on use of human embryos in cell research. *The New York Times,* p. A1.

Wade, N. (2000b, November 7). Teaching the body to heal itself; work on cell's signals fosters talk of a new medicine. *The New York Times,* p. F1.

Wade, N. (2001a, April 3). Findings deepen debate on using embryonic cells. *The New York Times,* p. F1.

Wade, N. (2001b, December 18). In tiny cells, glimpses of body's master plan. *The New York Times,* p. F1.

Wade, N. (2001c, April 27). Scientists report 2 major advances in stem-cell research. *The New York Times,* p. A21.

Wagner, W., & Kronberger, N. (2001). Killer tomatoes! Collective symbolic coping with biotechnology. In K. Deaux & G. Philgène (Eds.), *Representations of the social: Bridging theoretical traditions.* Malden, MA: Blackwell Publishers.

Walton, D. (2001). Persuasive definitions and public policy arguments. *Argumentation and Advocacy, 37,* 117–132.

Ward, M. (2000, April 24). UW-Madison cell research stems from curiosity about how replication works and what its benefits could be. *Milwaukee Journal Sentinel,* p. 1G.

Watt, F. M. (2001). Stem cell fate and patterning in mammalian epidermis. *Current Opinion in Genetics and Development, 11*(4), 410–417.

Watt, F. M., & Hogan, B. L. M. (2000). Out of Eden: Stem cells and their niches. *Science, 287,* 1427–1430.

Weaver, R. M. (1952). *The ethics of rhetoric.* Chicago: Henry Regnery.

Weaver, R. M. (1970). *Language is sermonic.* Baton Rouge: Louisiana State University Press.

Weingart, P. (2002). The moment of truth for science. *EMBO reports, 3*(8), 703–706.

Weiss, R. (1998, December 2). For Senate, "stem cell" advances revive an embryonic controversy. *The Washington Post,* p. A2.

Weiss, R. (2000a, April 19). Embryonic breakthroughs? Stem cell studies race ahead as U.S. policy languishes. *The Washington Post,* p. A1.

Weiss, R. (2000b, April 24). In cell "alchemy," an alternative to embryo studies. *The Washington Post,* p. A11.

Weiss, R. (2000c, August 15). Researchers transform bone marrow from adults. *The Washington Post,* p. A6.

Weiss, R. (2006, August 26). Critic alleges deceit in study on stem cells. *The Washington Post,* p. A02.

Weissman, I. L. (2000a). Stem cells: Units of development, units of regeneration, units of evolution. *Cell, 100,* 157–168.

Weissman, I. L. (2000b). Translating stem and progenitor cell biology to the clinic: Barriers and opportunities. *Science, 287*(5457), 1442–1446.

Weissman, I. L., Anderson, D. J., & Gage, F. H. (2001). Stem and progenitor cells: origins, phenotypes, lineage commitments, and transdifferentiations. *Annual Review of Cell and Developmental Biology, 17,* 387–403.

What Nancy Reagan's future holds. (2004). New York: CBS News.

Where the presidential candidates stand on the issue of stem cell research. (2004). New York: CBS News.

Whether stem cell research should become federally funded. (2001). New York: CBS News.

Wilcox, S. (2003). Cultural context and the conventions of science journalism: Drama and the contradiction in media coverage of biological ideas about sexuality. *Critical Studies in Media Communication, 20,* 225–247.

Williams, C., Alderson, P., & Farsides, B. (2001). Conflicting perceptions of the fetus: Person, patient, "nobody," commodity? *New Genetics and Society, 20*(3), 225–238.

Williams, R. (1983). *Keywords: A vocabulary of culture and society* (2nd ed.). London: Oxford University Press.

Wulf, G. G., Jackson, K. A., & Goodell, M. A. (2001). Somatic stem cell plasticity: Current evidence and emerging concepts. *Experimental Hematology, 29*(12), 1361–1370.

Wurmser, A. E., & Gage, F. H. (2002). Cell fusion causes confusion. *Nature, 416,* 485–487.

Xu, R.-H., Peck, R. M., Li, D. S., Feng, X., Ludwig, T., & Thomson, J. A. (2005). Basic FGF and suppression of DMP signaling sustain undifferentiated proliferation of human ES cells. *Nature Methods, 2,* 185–190.

Zarefsky, D. (1998). Definitions. In J. F. Klumpp (Ed.), *Argument in a time of change: Definitions, frameworks and critiques* (pp. 1-11). Annandale, VA: National Communication Association.

Zarefsky, D., Miller-Tutzauer, C., & Tutzauer, F. E. (1984). Reagan's safety net for the truly needy: The rhetorical uses of definition. *Central States Speech Journal, 35,* 113–119.

Zimmer, C. (2001). *Evolution: The triumph of an idea.* New York: Harper Collins.

Zitner, A. (1999, December 26). Debate looms over stem cell funds, research. *The Boston Globe,* p. A1.

Index